WHAT OTHERS ARE SAYING

It's No Biggie! is a gem. It is an insightful, extremely well-written, well-researched window into a long-neglected area. The book is interesting and practical beyond its target audience of professional educators. It will certainly help me to better serve my pediatric patients and their families. My thanks to Dr. Barboa and Ms. Datema for this important work!

Mark Ellis, M.D.

It's No Biggie! is an easy-to-read guidebook for teachers who wish to provide a successful learning environment for all of their young children, including those with characteristics of autism. Dr. Linda Barboa and Mary Lou Datema write from an extensive background of experience and their practical strategies will ensure increased growth and development for students in any early childhood classroom.

Peggy Reed, Ed.D.
Associate Professor of Early Childhood Education
Evangel University

Early intervention was one of the greatest things for our family. I learned how to communicate with my kids as well as how to teach them. Having teachers that are well educated about autism come alongside parents/families, is one of the greatest resource for a family that has just been given a diagnosis. When we drop our kids off with the teacher, we need to feel that they understand our kids and that they 'get it'. It really is *"No Biggie!"* This book is such a great resource for teachers that are feeling a bit overwhelmed in the classroom. *It's No Biggie!* is the book you want to put on your shelf after reading it through and refer back to it again and again as a refresher.

Shelli Allen
"ThatAutismMom.com"

Kids with autism can see the world in a different way, and it is important for teachers to understand that so they can help them. If teachers understand autism, it helps the student learn better and faster, and helps the teachers have an easier job.

Jaqi Bradshaw
Middle School Student on the Autism Spectrum

I highly recommend this book to early childhood teachers and to parents alike. This book starts with the basics of education and builds on that information to give the reader the solid foundation needed to teach special needs children, whether they have a formal diagnosis or not. The thing I love about this book is that it is a tool to help the teacher really enjoy each child—not just tolerate him. The authors provide real life scenarios and stories to put a face to the issues they discuss. They make the information interesting by relating it to children they have worked with. Every student in an education class should read this book.

Tina Steadman
Parent

This book should be required reading for all students who are preparing to be teachers. *It's No Biggie!* guides the reader by presenting the teacher's perspective, the parent's perspective, and most importantly, the child's perspective. As a parent, I truly wish this book had been available when my children were in preschool. As an education professional, I believe this book would benefit each and every early childhood teacher who is trying to make her classroom a better experience for all. *"It's No Biggie!"* is an easy read with practical suggestions to classroom problems.

Kristina Heth
Speech-Language Pathologist

As early childhood educators, we must be prepared to meet the needs of youngsters diagnosed with autism, as well as those with autism not yet identified. *It's No Biggie!* gives us the tools to meet the needs of those students and help them reach their maximum potential by providing proven intervention strategies that will reduce the social and language deficits typical of autism. I recommend this book to the seasoned, veteran teacher as well as the new teachers. Thanks to Ms. Datema and Dr. Barboa for meeting a real need by writing this book.

Sandy Nicholson
Early Childhood Teacher

Although my professional background is in nursing and counseling, I was never educated on autism. It wasn't until one of my own children started slipping away into that unknown world that I quickly became familiar with the disorder. What I wouldn't have given to have had this book at my fingertips during those first few years! We were incredibly blessed with devoted educators and therapists who were always available to answer questions and guide me in my quest to help our child. Not every parent is so fortunate. This book will fill a tremendous void for those desperate to help a child. Whether you are a school teacher, a parent, a preschool teacher, or anyone who works with children...the information the authors have provided is invaluable and a must read. You owe it to the children you encounter each day to make yourself as versed in ASD as possible.

Marcia N. Ellis, RN, BSN, MS

It's No Biggie!

Autism in the Early Childhood Classroom

Second Edition

DR. LINDA BARBOA

MARY LOU DATEMA

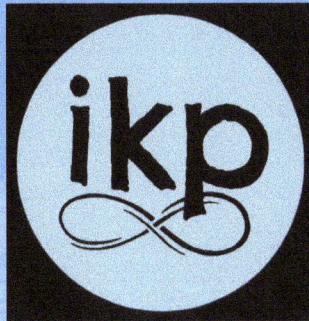

ikp

INFINITY KIDS PRESS

Kansas City

Acknowledgements

The authors would like to thank Mr. Muse Watson, (AKA Mike Franks, NCIS) for planting the initial seed which has bloomed into an amazing garden of gifts to the reader. Parents, teachers, and students with autism will benefit from his kindness for years to come in the collection of books he has inspired. We thank Sherry Wilson, Jennifer Cantrell, Dixie Love and family, and the Early Childhood Special Education Staff at Springfield Public Schools, Springfield, Missouri, for the many visual ideas and examples included in the book. Special thanks to teachers and therapists, Aubrey Smith Wilson, LaRissa Newman, Jean Lawson, Chrissy Spurlock, and Melissa Knetzer for sharing their excellent pictures and strategies; and for the beautiful spot art we thank Stacy Sheppard. Ben Datema is appreciated for his on the spot technical assistance. We want to acknowledge our beta readers Jan Luck and Sandy Nicholson for their input which certainly improved the quality of the book. We appreciate Amy Fink for her contribution to the foreword in this book. Our deepest gratitude we give to Goldminds Publishing for recognizing the value in this manuscript and their dedication to autism education.

About the Authors

Dr. Barboa holds degrees in speech pathology and audiology, communication sciences and disorders, psychology, and early childhood education. She is an experienced speech-language pathologist, with a background as a special education director, director of an autism center, and university professor. She has worked as an educator in America and Europe and has presented numerous programs to professionals across the country. Dr. Barboa has authored several books including *Stars in Her Eyes: Navigating the Maze of Childhood Autism*, which she wrote with Elizabeth Obrey. Her other books include *Autism—What Schools Are Missing: Voices for a New Path*, and a children's series about autism, based on the book *Albert is My Friend*. Dr. Barboa is the recipient of the Jefferson Award for Community Service.

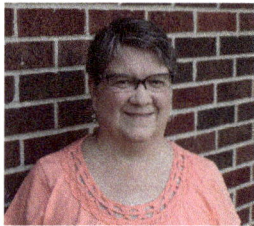

Mary Lou Datema began her teaching career at age 16, working in a local child care center after school.....for a dollar an hour. She now holds a Bachelor's degree in Elementary Education (early childhood) and a Master's degree in Reading as well as early childhood special education certification. Mary Lou has taught at the preschool, kindergarten and college levels in a variety of settings for over 40 years. She is currently an adjunct instructor at Ozarks Technical Community College. She has served in a variety of advisory capacities at the local and state level. She was named Teacher of the Year for the Springfield, Missouri school district in 2003. Mary Lou raised three boys on a steady diet of books, and now, in her spare time, she loves being a grandma and sharing her love of reading with her grandchildren.

Lovingly dedicated to
our families
by birth and by blessing

Table of Contents

PART FOUR -- RESOURCES

Introduction

Working with young children is a rewarding job, but it's also challenging, even on the best of days. Early childhood teachers work with a variety of abilities and behaviors and make hundreds of decisions daily that affect the lives of children. Every move you make and each word you utter will be studied and mimicked by little ones. The lessons they learn by observing your demeanor and attitude will have an effect on their formative years. As a teacher, having a bag of tricks that contains knowledge of child development as well as specific strategies to use in handling issues that arise is necessary.

We hope this book gives you a basic understanding of child development that will help you teach all those children who fall outside the "box" or along the autism spectrum, with or without a diagnosis. The basic behavioral concepts and strategies you will read about in this book will provide a foundational knowledge of child development. The more specific teaching tips will give you a variety of ways to work with those children who have additional challenges. When armed with knowledge of child development, an understanding of the autism spectrum, and good practical strategies for intervention, you will able to make your inclusive classroom a great place to be for everyone. It's no biggie!

Dr. Linda Barboa
Mary Lou Datema

"Early childhood inclusion embodies the values, policies and practices that support the right of every infant and young child and his or her family, regardless of ability, to participate in a broad range of activities and contexts as full members of families, communities, and society. The desired results of inclusive experiences for children with and without disabilities and their families include a sense of belonging and membership, positive social relationships and friendships, and development and learning to reach their full potential. The defining features of inclusion that can be used to identify high quality early childhood programs and services are access, participation and supports."

- Access - means providing a wide range of activities and environments for every child by removing physical barriers and offering multiple ways to promote learning and development.
- Participation - means using a range of instructional approaches to promote engagement in play and learning activities, and a sense of belonging for every child.
- Supports - refers to broader aspects of the system such as professional development, incentives for inclusion, and opportunities for communication and collaboration among families and professionals to assure high quality inclusion.

National Association for the Education of Young Children, April 2009 [1]

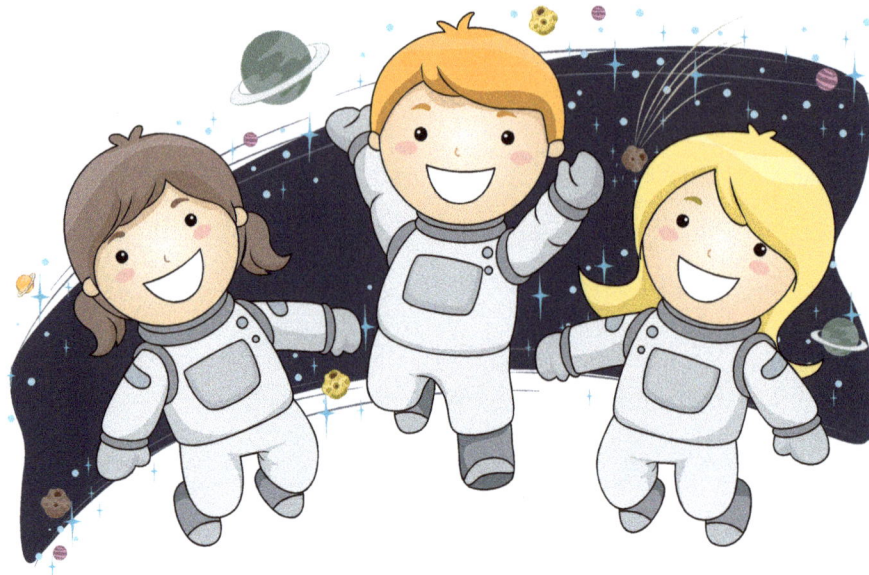

"I touch the future. I teach."
Christa McCauliffe, Teacher from the Space Shuttle Challenger, (1948-1986)

Foreword

"Teachers affect eternity; no one can tell where their influence stops." Like many educators, I came across this Henry Brooks Adams quote early in my teaching career. I can't remember how I discovered these words … a search for usable quotes during a late night push to finish a pedagogy paper, or perhaps it was an inspirational quote from a desk calendar. I don't remember where or how I happened upon those words, but I do remember the sense of gravity I felt when I read them and the profound way the words resonated within me.

I began my career as an early childhood educator thirteen years ago. Thirteen years sounds like a relatively short amount of time; however, I have seen a great deal of change during this time. One major area of change is the increasing prevalence of children with autism spectrum disorder. [2] This startling increase has helped bring to light the impact and importance of early intervention. Research tells us that no matter what the developmental disability or delay, that early intervention and detection are key because this is when the most impact can be made.

Allow me to introduce (or reintroduce) you, the reader, to the authors of *It's No Biggie! Autism in the Early Childhood Classroom*, Dr. Linda Barboa and Mary Lou Datema. Dr. Barboa has 45 years of experience, and Mary Lou Datema has 34 years of experience working in early childhood special education. They have worked with countless children with varying developmental disabilities and delays, and practiced early intervention strategies on a daily basis over the course of these years. This book is the tangible incarnation of their 79 years of combined experience.

It's No Biggie! is written specifically about autism; however, the information in this book can be applied to any classroom, even those without children with autism spectrum disorder. The book includes concepts and strategies for improving the physical classroom environment, effective teacher communication, teaching social skills, sensory processing, language development, social-emotional development, understanding and dealing with behaviors, and many more! Information for these concepts and strategies is given a personal touch with anecdotes and pictures from real classrooms. Key symbols can be found throughout the book with bullet points that summarize and restate key concepts. These key bullet points are wonderful for refresher reviews and quick reference. There is so much practical and useful information in this book—the personal stories, strategies, and interventions—that I recommend reading it with not only a highlighter, but a backup highlighter as well!

To paraphrase Henry Adams, like teachers, early intervention affects eternity. It positively influences the quality of life and futures of children with developmental disabilities and delays. "Affecting eternity" is an extraordinary responsibility, and as teachers, we reach into the future every day when we work with children. With their book and the invaluable information and guidance contained therein, Dr. Linda Barboa and Mary Lou Datema have managed to take some of the weight from that responsibility and, in doing so, have taught us that, "It's no biggie!"

Amy Fink, Early Childhood Educator

PART ONE
AUTISM BASICS

Chapter 1

The Teacher's Perspective
Keys to Understanding

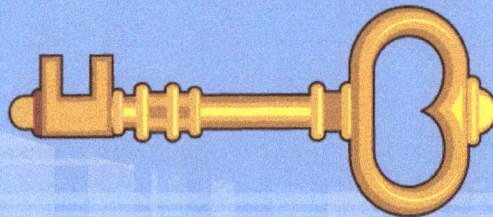

A few short decades ago, autism was a topic studied in college, but most teachers had never met a child with that diagnosis. If a school did happen to enroll a child with autism spectrum disorder, curious teachers would stop by that classroom, anxious to meet the new little friend and to see what autism really "looked like." At that point in history, those teachers could never have imagined nor predicted the explosion in incidence that would occur over the next few decades. There was no thought in their minds that in the coming years there would be children with autistic characteristics in virtually every classroom needing patient, educated, caring professionals to teach them. As of this printing, the Center for Disease Control estimates the prevalence of autism to be one in every 45 children, or about 2% of the children in the United States. Other countries give even higher estimates. Additionally, with each of those children comes parents or guardians seeking answers and guidance from professionals such as you.

Autism is a **neurobiological disorder** that occurs on a continuum and can range from mild to severe. Autism affects social interactions, communication and sensory processing. The cause of autism remains unknown, although a genetic component is suspected. Autism has not been proven to be caused by anything a parent did or did not do. Neither is it caused by lack of love or poor parenting skills. No definitive cause of autism has yet been found, although many suspected factors may contribute to the cause. The fact that no one knows the cause of autism leaves parents to wonder and guess. They may feel guilty as they wonder if something they did caused this. They may mentally point fingers at their spouse for some unknown action that may have caused it. The mystery of the cause may result in tensions in the home life, fueled by this guilt and blame. Teachers need to understand that autism affects not only the child, but the entire extended family, emotionally and financially.

Now, the incidence of autism is rising at an alarming rate, as shown in this graphic on the next page by the Center for Disease Control. [3] Even though this is the newest data released as of this publication, note that it is several years old. With the rate going up significantly every year, you can guess what the more realistic rate is currently.

Identified Prevalence of Autism Spectrum Disorder ADDM Network 2000-2023 Combining Data from All Sites				
Surveillance Year	Birth Year	Number of ADDM Sites Reporting	Prevalence per 1000 Children (Range)	This is about 1 in X children…
2000	1992	6	6.7 (4.5 - 9.9)	1 in 150
2004	1996	8	8.0 (4.6 – 9.8)	1 in 125
2008	2000	14	11.3 (4.8 – 21.2)	1 in 88
2012	2004	11	14.5 (8.2 - 24.6)	1 in 69
2016	2008	11	18.5 (18.0 – 19.1)	1 in 54
2020	2012	11	27.6 (23.1 – 44.9)	1 in 36

You may have students in your classroom with a diagnosis of autism. You may have students that you suspect may fall somewhere on the spectrum, but don't yet have a diagnosis. You may have some "quirky" kids who are just different, yet don't meet the criteria for a diagnosis. If you work with children who exhibit some of the characteristics of autism, you will be smart to learn to work with the challenges that autism presents.

Here are some common "red flags" of autism that you may see:

- delay in or lack of functional communication
- avoids eye contact
- unresponsiveness to people; people are treated more like objects
- lack of joint attention; the child doesn't follow your finger when you point
- repetitive play routines; lining up objects; repeating one specific activity over and over

- difficulty making social connections
- resistant to change
- follows rigid routines
- unusual self-stimulatory or self-injurious behaviors
- skill development doesn't follow typical developmental patterns

Characteristics you may see in children on the autism spectrum are individualized and widely varied. Some children on the autism spectrum are nonverbal and non-responsive to most things (and people) in their environment. At the age of four, Matthew was nonverbal, lacked play skills, and was unable to toilet or bathe independently. Matthew did not respond to his name or show affection to family members. He could stand at the bathroom sink and let the water run into his hands for hours. When he wanted the CD player turned on with his favorite songs, he would bang on the table beside it. This was the only activity he ever requested. Some children are much higher functioning, and it may take much longer for a casual observer to pick up on red flags. Brennan was very verbal and had an amazing vocabulary for naming objects. By age four, he could read at a second grade level, but he still had difficulty answering simple questions, carrying on a conversation or playing with another child.

These behaviors fall along a **spectrum**. Some children with autism are completely nonverbal and non-responsive. Some children with autism are very verbal, very bright, and deal with milder impairments in communication. Those in the field who work with children on the autism spectrum will tell you very quickly, "If you've met one child with autism, you've met one child with autism," a phrase coined by Steven Mark Shore. A child on the spectrum may be able to give you very detailed information on whales, but not be able to answer a simple social question such as, "How are you?" A child on the spectrum may talk *at* you rather than *with* you, may have a hard time seeing the point of view of another person, and may not enjoy the toys and activities most children enjoy. There are often difficulties with social and play skills. A child with autism may show very advanced skills in some areas paired with significant deficits in other skills areas.

If you notice one or more of the red flags listed above apply to a child you teach, it is not your responsibility or prerogative to give a diagnosis to the parent. Even if the parent asks your opinion as to whether or not the child has autism, you are not qualified to **diagnose**. You can, however, tell the parent what specific behaviors you notice in the class and suggest they discuss these behaviors with the pediatrician on the next visit. Just as you would not diagnose any medical illness, the teacher does not diagnose autism. It is a medical diagnosis, not an educational label. You and the parent give your specific findings to the proper medical practitioners who can legally make this diagnosis. Give your list of concerns to the parent who can discuss this with the child's pediatrician. For legal reasons, teachers do not share their information with any outside person, including those in the medical field, without written permission from the parent.

KEY POINTS

- Even though every child is unique, there is a set of common characteristics identified in many people with autism.
- Autism is a spectrum disorder, meaning that the characteristics and skills fall along a wide range.
- Teachers must get written permission from the parent or guardian to share information about a child.

A commonly identified characteristic of children with ASD is **repetitive movement**. This may take the form of **ritualistic movements**. Rituals may be stimulating to the child or may enable him to feel in control. They may give him a sense of comfort. An example of a child demonstrating a ritual is Jaden, who turns the light switch on and off repeatedly. Rituals may revolve around food, clothing, toys, daily activities, or behaviors.

Some rituals get quite complicated, such as when Remi's family is leaving the house. Before she will leave, she flips the light switch several times, claps a half dozen times, laughs, then opens and closes the door three times. Only then will she leave without a loud protest. Children who have better communication skills can sometimes explain the root of the ritual. When Kimmy was young, she balked at going through the doorway following another person.

She would turn sideways, duck, hold her breath and slide through with her eyes closed. This odd ritual was more pronounced when she did not particularly like the person. In later years as her communication improved, she explained that she was afraid that she might get another person's "stuff" on her if she went through the doorway too soon after that person.

Other seemingly odd behaviors may serve the purpose of **self-stimulation**. These actions are commonly referred to in a shortened form, as "self-stimming." When a child is in need of stimulation and is not receiving the amount needed, he will begin to create stimulation for himself. You may see a child spinning, rocking, or hand flapping. There may be any number of activities used by the child to serve this purpose. It may be finger flicking, head banging, laughing, running or shouting. Another reason a child may "self-stim" is actually to calm himself. He may have learned to use a certain behavior as a self-calming behavior when he is overly excited. This might look a little different for every child.

Children on the spectrum like rules. It comforts them to know the rule in any situation. It is a structure in which they thrive. They may be very upset if others don't follow the rules. Remember this refers to the rule as *they* perceive it. If they are told that there is a school rule not to talk in the library, and then the librarian begins to read to the children, they may get upset because she is not following the rule. They will be highly distressed when other children do not follow the rules. If you have a classroom rule that children should, "Stay on your carpet square during circle time," but then a fire drill happens and they all have to get up, he may be upset at being forced to break a rule. If the rule is to walk on the right side of the hall when you go to recess, but the right side of the wall has been freshly painted, and is wet and the class has to walk on the left side, he may be upset. Anderson became upset when his school box broke and his teacher put his things in a small cardboard shoe box. The rule stated that every student should carry his school box to art, and the replacement box was not a "school box."

Children on the autism spectrum have difficulty with social and conversational skills.

Charles loved sharks, and could tell you everything about sharks, whether you were interested or not. Because this was a conversational comfort zone for Charles, he tended to talk about sharks a lot when meeting new people. He resisted anyone trying to change the topic and talked *at* people rather than *to* them. Charles was always in charge of the conversation, and had trouble responding to a variety of topics, or give and take in conversations. Charles simply couldn't understand why everybody wasn't as interested in sharks as he was. Nor did he care. He simply continued to push the topic of sharks through his one-way conversations as others carried on more social conversations despite his inappropriate contributions. Like Charles, a child may be obsessed with a given topic and stick to that topic no matter what direction the conversation is taking around him.

Others, however, struggle to stay on topic. You, as the teacher, will continue to guide him back to the topic at hand. In this way he will learn to maintain a conversation.

Children on the autism spectrum often show difficulties with play skills. Seth had a hard time engaging with his environment. His grandma called him a "good boy" because he would sit quietly on the couch for hours at a time. Seth was nonverbal and did not have any functional play skills, but would push a toy train back and forth over and over. He never acknowledged his caregivers with hellos or goodbyes but would pull on an adult hand to guide them to the refrigerator for juice.

Children on the autism spectrum may display what we call "**splinter skills**." They may display some areas of very advanced development, paired with areas of average or below average development. This can be displayed in some unusual interests. Josh had always loved numbers. He could add four and five digit numbers very quickly in his head, and had memorized the telephone numbers of family members, but was unable to answer simple questions. Some of those advanced skills may be misinterpreted by those around the child. A child with autism may be "**hyperlexic**" and seem to be reading far above expectation. In reality he may just have a splinter skill of "word calling," with no idea of what he is actually reading. The same may be true of numbers. He may display a phenomenal mathematical ability, but not be able to count the four pegs you are holding in front of him. Some children with autism may display some very advanced, very specific skills, but when you look at the skills more deeply, large gaps in knowledge and understanding are present.

Four-year-old Randy had some functional communication, but was able to read at a second grade level. He was unable to comprehend or explain what he read, but had mastered the letter/sound system at the age of three. Even though he was able to read words, he had limited comprehension of what he read. In the classroom setting, he relied on the use of pictures to tell him the schedule of activities and the class rules. Randy **perseverated**, or fixated on letters and numbers. He could stand in front of the alphabet poster in the classroom and recite the alphabet for the entire morning. The teacher had to remove the poster from the classroom.

Izzy, six years old, was seen as having behavior problems when she went to speech therapy sessions. Izzy was nonverbal and unable to explain her frustrations to the speech-language pathologist. When she came to speech, rather than sitting nicely in a chair, she immediately began tearing the pretty, colorful scrambled alphabet decorations off the wall. When her mother visited the therapy session, she quickly saw that Izzy was merely trying to put the randomized, chaotic alphabet letters into order, rather than leaving them in the scrambled order they were arranged in on the cute wall decoration. Because Izzy was nonverbal it did not occur to the therapist that the child was actually trying to put the alphabet into the correct order.

Children on the spectrum may be obsessed with routine. Dante came back a little late from speech therapy, and realized his class had already gone to lunch, and were just finishing up going through the lunch line. He became very upset when he realized he was out of his usual routine of going through the line with his peers. He refused to go through the line himself without his peers, and was unable to calm himself or to understand it was okay to do things a little differently that day.

Children on the spectrum may have unusual interests. Parker, a twelve-year-old boy on the spectrum, had a particular interest in security systems. He displayed an astounding knowledge of different systems and how they work. Store employees always enjoyed answering his security questions, until the depth of knowledge he had began to make them just a little uncomfortable.

Children on the spectrum may not understand typical humor. Jeff, an early childhood student, went to the end of the year assembly at his elementary school with his class. Part of the festivities included a dunk tank for the principal. Jeff didn't understand why this was fun, or why students were laughing when the principal was dunked. That was not funny at all to him.

Sometimes children on the spectrum have unusual fears. Steven was terrified of butterflies, and would try to hide under the teacher's skirt when a butterfly came near. After trying to introduce him to dead (not moving) butterflies, and finding that was not a problem, the teacher realized it was the erratic movements of the butterfly that frightened him.

🗝 KEY POINTS

- Children with autism often display behaviors which are rituals to them.
- They are comforted by rules because rules make the world predictable for them.
- People on the spectrum have difficulty with social skills and social communication.
- Children with ASD may have some skills, known as splinter skills, which are far above the rest of their skills.
- They may be obsessed with keeping a routine.
- Unusual fears may be noted.

On the higher functioning end of the autism spectrum is **Asperger's Syndrome**. Asperger's Syndrome has recently been swept under the umbrella of autism, for purposes of official medical terminology. However, for those who are striving to provide an educational program on a daily basis, you need to understand the specific characteristics of those children on the autism spectrum characterized as having Asperger's. Asperger's is distinctly different from the main categorization of high functioning autism. While the two categories do share some common characteristics, there are observable differences. Children who have autism have a distinctively higher level of **receptive language** than **expressive language**. Those two skill sets are more equal for a child with Asperger's. A child with Asperger's usually does not have a language deficit, cognitive delay or delay in many self-help skills. He will, however, show impairments in social interactions, and in some activities of daily living. A child with Asperger's may display restricted, repetitive and stereotyped patterns of behavior that we identify as autistic behaviors. The new medical terminology, used by insurance companies, groups all of the points of the spectrum into one classification, "autism spectrum disorder." However, you will still find the term "Asperger's," one segment of autism, to be a commonly used term. You will also hear various affectionate terms for people who show these characteristics, such as the term, "Aspies."

Although some characteristics of autism are shared to an extent, the range of abilities, and combinations of abilities is endless. When you look at each child, recognize that each is exactly that—a unique child with abilities and challenges. You have accepted a job to teach children, and that means teaching *every child* in the way that he or she can best learn. By reading this book, you are taking the first step toward fulfilling the huge commitment you have agreed to. Congratulations for being willing to learn and succeed. It's no biggie!

KEY POINTS

- Asperger's Syndrome is one classification of autism, characterized by social difficulties.
- Children with Asperger's typically have good communication skills.
- Each child with autism is unique.

Sensory Processing

Autism can be marked by disturbances in how sensory information is processed. We all tolerate sensory input in different ways and in differing amounts. Our individual variations in sensory tolerance are not a problem until they begin to interfere with daily life, and this is true of individuals on the autism spectrum as well. Some children on the spectrum have a very small sensory "cup," and it doesn't take much for them to become overwhelmed by sensory input, and for their imaginary cup to feel very full very soon. In contrast, other children have huge cups and can never seem to find enough sensory input in their environments to meet their needs. Sensory issues are very real and need to be handled accordingly. These triggers can make or break any classroom activity. Learning to understand and respect the fears and discomforts is the first step along your path to resolving the problem.

You will have students in your classroom who are sensory seekers and others who are sensory avoiders. These children are not behaving this way to defy you as a teacher, or to get attention; they are trying to meet their own basic sensory needs. Sensory disturbances, sometimes referred to as **sensory processing disorders**, are common in children on the autism spectrum, but can also be found in children who don't have an autism diagnosis, or any diagnosis at all. To be truly considered a "disorder" the behaviors must be frequent, persistent, and interfere to some extent with daily functioning. However, paying close attention to any child who seems to have sensory issues and making some simple changes benefits everybody, diagnosis or not.

When our bodies process sensory information, this is called **sensory integration**. Our brains organize and analyze the sensory input, and this results in our bodies functioning better.

For example, Anjie was a very sensory-seeking child and loved paint, shaving cream, mud and anything else she could delightedly smear on her arms. Going outside to be pushed in the swing was very rewarding for her. In contrast, Emma was very sensory avoiding and would shriek and run away any time the teacher introduced paint or shaving cream. In working with students on the spectrum, you will find endless variations in how these children react to sensory input. You may find a child who craves tactile (touch) experiences, but is very sensitive to loud noises, or one who has a very small cup when it comes to taste and smell, but a *huge* cup when it comes to the need for movement. Being good observers of your students, their likes and dislikes, will teach you much about the effects of sensory input.

It is important for you, as the teacher, to acknowledge the effect that various stimuli are having on a particular child and how you can be prepared for his responses. The different stimulations that are constantly bombarding a person are known as sensory input. These stimuli can be received through your hearing, your vision, touch or taste, or smell. Those are the senses we normally learn about in school. There are a couple more senses that may be affected by autism. One of those is the **vestibular** sense and the other is the sense of **proprioception**. A good teacher will consider all seven of these senses when teaching a child on the spectrum.

A child can be overly sensitive (**hypersensitive**) or under-sensitive (**hyposensitive**) in each of the seven senses discussed here. To complicate factors, he may be hypersensitive to a stimuli one day and hyposensitive the next. For example, a child may seem not to even hear the doorbell one day, but the next day may scream in pain when the doorbell rings.

🔑 KEY POINTS

- Children may be overly sensitive or under-sensitive in one or more of the senses.
- You will have students in your classroom who are sensory seekers and others who are sensory avoiders.
- It is important to acknowledge the effect that various stimuli are having on a particular child.

Most people consider sight to be one of their most highly valued senses. A tremendous amount of information is gathered through our visual sense if it is working properly for us. While visual acuity refers to how well a person can actually see, visual perception refers to how the stimulus is processed by the brain. The same applies to each of the other senses as we discuss them here. Inadequate processing of any type of stimuli can cause avoidance behaviors or over-excitement in your students.

Many children are hypersensitive to light and want to wear their hats or their sunglasses to soften the light that may actually hurt their eyes. On the other hand, children with issues related to vision may actually be driven to stare at lights or at the sun. Other visual problems may be difficulty in shifting their gaze from one object to another, or difficulty with eye contact. Some children may get easily exhausted when presented with multiple visual stimuli. Others may begin to squint to reduce the incoming stimuli. Nathan was very sensitive to light, so he would squint his eyes in a way that actually looked like he was winking. People found that little facial contortion to be endearing and thought it was cute, but it was actually a signal of distress.

Visual preferences may affect the child in ways such as limiting the clothing he wears or the toys he will play with. The visual presentation of foods offered to him maybe affected by his color preference.

Most typical children receive large amounts of information through the sense of hearing. Children with autism may have auditory sensitivities. They may perceive noises as much louder than they really are, or they may not even notice a particular auditory stimulus. One little boy walked around the school with crayons sticking out of his ears. This was his attempt to block out the noises that disturbed him. Some children cover their ears when music or other sounds are presented. They are trying to muffle it to bring down the volume. When children are subjected to sounds that are uncomfortable to them, it may result in unwanted behaviors. A behavior you may see in children with auditory sensitivity is hiding under tables or chairs when things seem to them to be chaotic.

Sometimes a child with autism will exhibit random verbalizations. He may hum or produce a chanting type of sound or repeat words seemingly just to himself. These noises are sometimes an effort to mask outside noises or voices which are bothering him.

Other children may actually be drawn to loud noises. Some may speak in a loud voice or yell because that is how they perceive the sound level around them to be. When a child is hypersensitive to sounds, it can interfere with his learning. As you are trying to teach him in the classroom, your clear, crisp voice may be drowned out by a sound of the heater, or the voice of a teacher in a room down the hall.

Tactile sensitivity refers to the sense of touch. A child may scream when he gets his face washed. Hair brushing may bring great pain. He may despise touching certain textures. On the other hand, he may crave feeling textures. As he walks down the hall, he may run his hand along the wall, delighting in the feel of the textured wall. He may take comfort in carrying a stuffed toy to rub or a piece of silky cloth, depending on the feeling he craves. He may hug too tightly or too roughly.

A child may demonstrate tactile sensitivity to something as light as air. The temperature of the air may affect his ability to function. A child who continually strips off his clothing may be reacting to an increased body temperature, or he could be sensitive to the feeling of the material against his skin. You will need to be a detective to determine what sensitivity is affecting a behavior. Other children may come to school wearing multiple layers of clothing and not want to remove their coats. They crave that tactile pressure. Children who fit into this category may benefit from the services of an occupational therapist who may suggest the use of weighted vests or weighted blankets to meet their needs. Sometimes the desire to constantly touch others or the choice to avoid touch is related to the tactile sensitivity of the child. Many children who have tactile sensitivity to touch tolerate it much better when presented as a firm touch, rather than a feathery light touch. Another suggestion when working with tactile sensitive children is to verbally prepare them for the touch so that it does not send them into a tailspin. An example of this would be, "Jax, I am going to move your hand to show you how to zip this coat."

Distorted tactile sensitivities explains why many children with autism may not feel pain as others do. They may not even seem to notice something that would be painful to another person, but may be extremely sensitive to a slight touch and scream in pain.

Another behavior you may see when children are craving tactile stimulation is hiding or crawling into tight spaces. They might continually make little tents or wrap themselves in blankets.

If your child has sensitivity related to taste, this might manifest as hypo or hyper sensitivity, just as with the auditory and visual senses. The hypersensitive child may refuse to eat any macaroni and cheese except that made by mom, and notice any subtle difference in taste. He may be able to tell if you bought the generic or name brand crackers and may point out the difference to you. If you learn that a particular child is hyposensitive (not very sensitive) to tastes, be diligent about keeping substances out of his reach. He may drink the bottle of paint that is sitting on the table, or a spray bottle of window cleaner if he can get his hands on it. He does not taste the difference between various substances, and is likely to eat or drink something toxic if it is in his field of vision. To him, bleach may taste the same as water. **Pica** is a disorder characterized by a compulsion to eat non-edible items, such as dirt or paint chips from the wall. If Pica is not carefully managed, it can lead to dental problems or medical issues. James constantly chewed the tires on toy cars until he loosened the rubber and ate it. This resulted in lifelong problems with his teeth. A group called We Are Teachers recently posted on Facebook that teaching is the only profession where we find ourselves saying, "We don't lick the pencil sharpener."

The sense of smell varies from person to person. This difference is magnified in children with autism. A child may actually despise the smell of flowers or perfume, or he may love it. Many of these children like to sniff the hair or the arms of those around them. Their sense of smell may be highly acute and they smell things that the rest of us do not smell. They are often upset by the smell of the teacher's breath, especially if it has a distinct odor, such as coffee. One teacher complained that on some days Max stood way too close when he talked to her, seeming not to understand personal space. Other days he stood way back, turning his head to the side and she could barely hear him when they had a conversation. When she asked him about it, he told her honestly that some days her breath stinks like coffee, but other days it smells good, like peppermint. Another child explained that when the teacher's breath stinks it is so distracting to him that he cannot hear what she is talking about.

A sense which you may not be so familiar with is the **vestibular** sense. This refers to the feeling of your body in relation to the earth. You may have children in your class who continually fall out of their chairs. You may have a child who feels the wall as he walks down the hall. That may be to help him keep his balance or his point of reference. These kids may be clumsy or appear to be off balance. Kids who crave this stimulation will want to climb and jump. If he is hypersensitive, he may fear stairs. He might avoid fast moving activities because that movement makes him feel nauseated. Ella hated any playground activity in which her feet did not touch the ground, and found any climbing or swinging activities very frightening.

Proprioception is another sense that may be new to you, as we don't learn much about it in school. This is the sense that gives us information about where our bodies are in space. This is how we know to duck our heads when we get into a car, or to turn sideways when we pass through a tight space. Children who are hyposensitive in the realm of proprioception may bump into others without realizing why. They may play too roughly, or appear to be awkward.

Interoception is the understanding of what is happening within one's body. The body sends messages to the brain signaling such sensations as hunger, sleepiness, pain, nausea, thirst, and bathroom needs. Children with autism may not perceive and understand these signals in a typical way. They may display inappropriate laughter or crying. They might have eating or sleeping disturbances. Typically, messages from the brain tell a person to eat, sleep, put on a coat, or use the restroom. Children on the spectrum may have difficulty understanding what their body is telling them, therefore accurate reporting of their internal states by be difficult. The teacher must understand that the child may get erroneous signals from their own body receptors. Interoceptive sensations may be very confusing for individuals affected by autism.

Although many sensory characteristics are shared to some extent, the range of sensitivities and sensory needs is endless.

🔑 KEY POINTS

- We all have sensory differences, but the differences in children with autism may be more noticeable and interfere more with daily life.
- Many behaviors are driven by differences in sensory sensitivity, as children seek or avoid the stimuli in order to find the balance their body craves.

Communication

Reaction to sensory stimuli is just one important component of autism. Another important aspect to understand is the struggle these children face with communication. Communication is the most important skill that humans develop. Your ability to survive in life depends on your ability to communicate. Likewise, your survival in the classroom will be linked to your ability to communicate effectively with students, their parents, and other professionals. Daniel Webster once said, "If all my possessions were taken from me with one exception, I would choose to keep the power of communication, for by it I would soon regain all the rest."[4] When you sharpen your own communication abilities all of your other teaching skills will improve. Life in the classroom will become easier and more enjoyable.

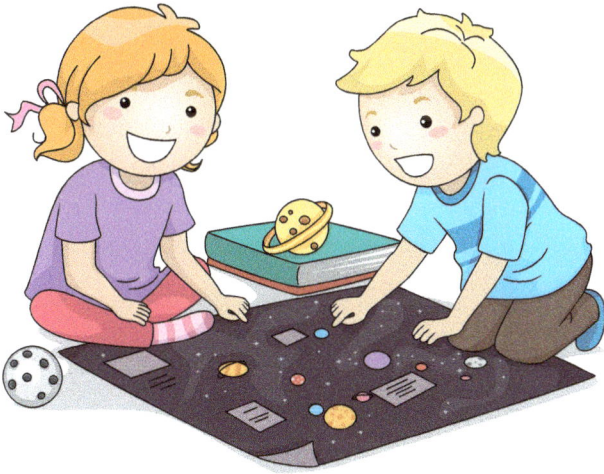

Communication is divided into two skills- the ability to understand what is presented by others, or **receptive language**, and the ability to make your thoughts known, or **expressive language**. The majority of children understand more than they can express. This is especially true of children who have autism. A child may understand what you are saying in front of him, even though he cannot speak at that level. Be certain that the things you say within his hearing range are meant for his ears. A child who hears negative things about himself, even if he cannot talk, will likely act out in another form.

Expressive language is language a child can produce himself. If you have a child with classic autism in your class, expect delayed or even absent expressive language. Many other developmental disabilities are characterized by expressive challenges. This is important for you to know because a lack of expressive language is often the root of frustration and leads to unwanted behaviors. If a child lacks language, his behaviors become his way of expressing himself. This is why it is so important for you to provide him with some basic communication tools. Expressive language may be either spoken, written or signed. If a child is unable to make his wants and needs known orally, but can learn to perform simple sign language to let you know what he needs, the child will stay more relaxed and more able to learn. As time goes by, you will use that manual sign to bridge the gap to the spoken word. A speech-language pathologist can help you with communication needs. If you do not know what SLP serves the qualifying students in your program, contact the local public school. They can normally guide you to services provided by the state or by the public school system, or help you find some teacher resources. There are modifications you can make in your teaching which will facilitate communication between you and the children. The SLP can assist you in those skills.

When you speak to your class, keep your vocabulary and your sentence structure simple. If you use vocabulary that is over their heads, they will only guess what you are saying. They will lose interest quickly. Imagine going to a lecture where you don't understand what the presenter is talking about because he uses big, technical words that are unfamiliar to you. You would quickly become mentally lost and stop listening altogether. Keep kids engaged by speaking to them in short, simple sentences and by using vocabulary they can understand. In your teaching, introduce them to new vocabulary by explaining what those words mean.

Another mistake that parents and teachers make when speaking to young children is to expect action from an indirect request. For example, if you say to a child, "Your face is dirty," he does not automatically translate this to the fact that he needs to go wash his face. To be effective, be more direct and say, "Go wash your face now."

Words or phrases that have multiple meanings present an additional challenge. Children need to be taught that words may have more than one meaning. A friend told us that as she was preparing her Thanksgiving dinner she realized she needed to insert the table leaves to extend the length of the table. She asked the kids to go to the storage area and get the *leaves* for the table. When she came into the dining room a few minutes later, she found a pile of autumn *leaves* in the middle of the table.

Another teacher once described her experience trying to teach basic concepts. One day she was showing pictures designed to show the difference between the concepts of *light* and *heavy*. One picture showed a man carrying a *light* suitcase and the other showed a man carrying a *heavy* suitcase. The children agreed that one suitcase looked *heavy*, but protested that the other did not have a *light* on it.

Another example is a boy named James who asked the teacher if they were going outside for recess. When she replied, "Yes, dear," he got upset. He told her that he is a *boy*, not a *deer*, and demanded, "Don't call me an animal!"

Phrases, as well as single words, might have multiple meanings. A mother shared with us a story of her sons playing with a little toy car on the table during dinner. She told the boys to "Knock it off!" She couldn't scold them when the car went flying to the floor after that directive, as they thought they were doing what she told them to do. Be aware of the many meanings a word or phrase might have, and say exactly what you mean.

The same is true with idioms. It is difficult for many children to understand figures of speech. Their thinking is very literal. They assume you mean what you say. If you tell these children, "It is raining cats and dogs," don't be surprised if they actually expect to see cats and dogs falling from the sky. If you tell them, "I've got a frog in my throat," they may fearfully ask how a frog got into your throat.

After a particularly successful language class Miss Susan praised her class. "You guys are really on fire today." They jumped up and ran screaming down the hall thinking that they were actually on fire. It took several hours to get them to really calm down. She needed to explain the meaning of that phrase to them. A few months later, one of them happily announced he is "on fire today." He explained that this does not mean he is *really* on fire, rather that he is doing a good job.

Be aware that prepositions can be confusing to early learners. Does, "Put the toys *up*." mean the same thing to a little one as "Put the toys *away*"? Likely not. Giving that first directive could mean that you find a child holding his blocks up in the air. Learn to monitor your speech so that you say what you actually mean. The main point to remember in your communication is that this population thinks in very literal thoughts. They take what you say literally. Abstract thinking is difficult for all young children, and especially so for those with autism. This struggle often continues into adulthood.

In addition to prepositions, you may find challenges in the understanding and use of pronouns. Some of the pronoun confusion may be the result of a lack of the concept of "self." If you ask Jax, "What is your name?" he may answer, "Your name is Jax." He may confuse the pronouns to use with inanimate objects. If you ask Emma where her cookie is, she may answer, "I ate her."

Children with autism often have difficulty answering questions and will require your patient guidance to learn this skill. Some sentences only require a single word to answer. These questions are much simpler for the child to answer. Questions that begin with the words "who, what, where, or when" can often be answered with one word. To help the child move forward in his language development, ask open-ended questions. Open-ended questions are questions that require more than one word to answer. Open-ended questions usually start with the words "how or why" and require more thought from the child. To answer an open-ended question requires more complex sentences from the child. This will take time, but each day you can help the child move toward this goal.

Every day in your classes you will promote the development of language skills in a variety of ways. As you go through your daily routine, this is a vital component to the success of your children. People communicate in many ways and speech is just one of those choices. Your goal when teaching children with special needs may be to teach them to talk. However, that is not always the most immediate goal. There are many forms of communication a child may use to communicate his wants and needs. The important thing is for the early learner to develop a way to express himself. This may be through words, or it may begin with gestures.

As early childhood teachers, we find ourselves constantly telling our little ones, "Use your words." Some of your students will have more than adequate words to express their wants and needs; some will not. Make sure before you expect a high level of verbal communication to solve problems and express needs appropriately that your student actually has the skills to be able to do so. You may have to help **scaffold** them through some verbal processes as they learn. You may have children in your class who do not have the ability to express their most basic needs. A child who does not have a basic form of communication will be frustrated, angry, and will likely become a behavior problem in an inclusive class. As the teacher, you must find the way to decrease this frustration before real learning can begin.

KEY POINTS

- Lack of expressive language is often the root of frustration and results in unwanted behaviors.
- A speech-language pathologist (speech therapist) can guide you in helping children with communication difficulties.

When you are communicating with a child on the spectrum, do not make promises or make any statements that he may consider to be a promise. If you make a strong statement that the child considers to be a promise, and then a situation comes along that creates a change in what you told him, this will upset the child tremendously, and he will have trouble trusting you from that point forward. If you tell your class that the group will always have lunch at 11:00, then one day the schedule gets interrupted for any reason, these children will be unduly upset. Likewise, you might tell them the school has a rule stating that when you go out to the playground you must use the door on the right hand side because other children are entering through the left side. Then, one day the right hand side of the door is broken and they must go out through the left side. This can precipitate a small crisis.

Another aspect of communication that is unique to this population is that they tend to not understand pointing. The whole concept of pointing to something must be taught to these children. This is part of the interaction we call "joint attention."

Many aspects of communication that typical children learn just by observing the people in their environment need to be actually *taught* to children with autism. They do not read body language, nor do they naturally interpret facial expressions. In fact, they may find facial expressions totally meaningless and even distracting. If a child is being scolded, he may giggle and laugh because he finds your "angry face" funny. He may think that it is amusing that when you get annoyed, your mouth gets small and round, and your eyes get bigger. Rather than paying attention to the correction, he is only looking at the funny face you are making. Luckily, with patience, these critical communication skills can be taught.

A common characteristic of the speech of children with autism spectrum disorder is **echolalia**. They may repeat a sound, a word or phrase they have just heard or it may crop up much later. It may pop out of their mouths in a single situation or they may perseverate and it will become a catch phrase they use daily, or even hourly. When Timmy was fourteen, he repeated the phrase, "Two weeks" continually, followed by a smile and a demonic laugh. Evan would often repeat the phrase, "This is terrible, just terrible," that he had learned from a Winnie the Pooh video. His mother was quick to point out to the classroom teacher that this was non-functional, repetitive, echolalic speech, and didn't mean things in her classroom were really terrible at all.

Sometimes the echolalia actually seems like part of the conversation. If you say to Alexa, "What is your name?" She will answer, "Your name." If you ask Owen, "Do you want to paint?" He will answer, "Paint" whether he really wants to paint, or not. The reply he gives is not really an answer to the question, as he is just echoing the last word of the sentence.

This is different from the "bababa" type of babbling verbalized by a baby as he learns to talk. The baby's repetition of sounds has a value, in that he is practicing and exploring new sounds. Echolalia is not usually considered to be productive. Sometimes it is quite inappropriate. When seven-year-old Izzy hears a baby cry, she mimics the sound, then laughs in delight. The parents of the child who is crying are generally not amused. Echolalia normally does not lead to useful language skills.

However, there are times when the echolalia does serve a function. If a child learns to mimic a word or phrase that can be used to meet their wants or needs, or to give information, it can serve a purpose. Timmy was not verbal enough to produce a spontaneous social greeting, but when he entered the classroom each morning, he would look at the teacher, Miss Mims, and repeat a phrase from the old Leave it to Beaver reruns he liked to watch, "Good morning, Miss Landers" or a phrase from the Popeye cartoon, "Ahoy, Matey!"

Echolalia can either be immediate, with the child repeating what he has just heard, or it can be delayed, popping out days or even weeks later. It can be a sound, a word or a phrase. Children can even memorize complete movies and repeat the script line for line. This is known as scripting. We may be amazed and think the child is brilliant because he can repeat such complicated works. However, the problem is that when he fills his communication with meaningless echolalia or scripting it interferes with his ability to learn and communicate functionally.

KEY POINTS

- Simple vocabulary and sentence structure help children with communication issues understand.
- Children on the spectrum need you to keep meanings clear.
- Inclusive words such as "always" and "never" can cause problems because they will be taken quite literally.
- Children on the spectrum may not understand body language, including pointing.
- Speech may be characterized by echolalia and scripting that is not functional.

Social Skills

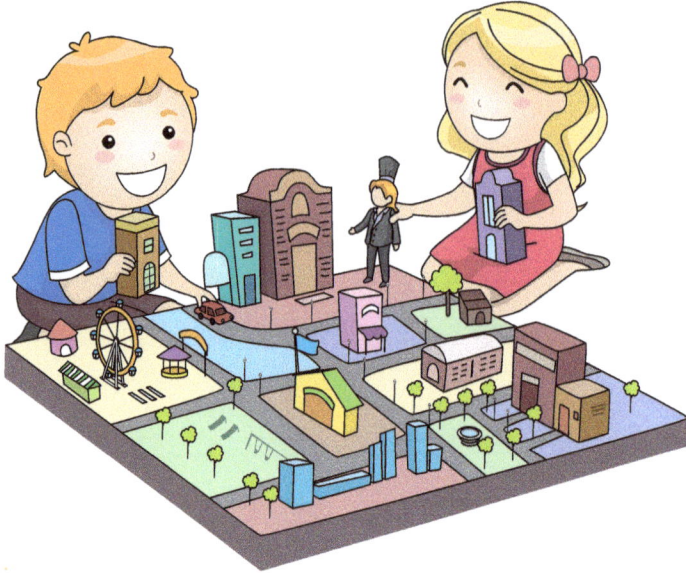

Children on the autism spectrum face many social challenges. Most typical children are motivated by the desire to please the adults in their lives, and to fit in socially with peers. They learn socially acceptable behavior by watching others, imitating what they do, and taking pride in the pleased reactions of others when they do the socially acceptable, "correct" thing. Children on the spectrum are often not very interested in fitting in with peers. Our friend Seth, discussed earlier, preferred sitting alone on the couch to playing with peers or with toys. Randy was interested in the alphabet chart on the wall, but not in making friends in his new classroom. They may choose to play alone as opposed to interacting with others, so social rewards might not work well, and time away from the group is not seen as a negative. However, some children on the autism spectrum may crave social connections but have difficulty understand how to make those connections happen.

As early childhood teachers, we work hard to build relationships with our students, and it can be very frustrating and confusing to work with a child who doesn't want a hug from you, is not eager to please you, and won't even make eye contact. Social praise may be meaningless to him. Failure to respond to your praise is not meant to be a personal affront. It's about how that child's brain works and not about you. It means that the incidental learning that takes places for most kids just by being in a school setting or being around others will not be present for kids on the spectrum. It may involve more teaching that is very specific to social skills.

Children with autism have trouble seeing the point of view of another person. They may not understand that other people have wants and needs just like they do. They are often unable to see the perspective of another person in games or at play. This affects social conventions in a negative way. If a child cannot see things from another person's point of view, it becomes impossible for him to feel empathy for that person. It affects his desire to take turns or to be socially appropriate, to be kind or comforting others.

10 THINGS EVERY CHILD WITH AUTISM WANTS YOU TO KNOW

1.	I am first and foremost a child. Autism is just one aspect of my character.	6.	It's hard for me to tell you what I need when I don't know the words to say it.
2.	Ordinary sights, sounds and touches of everyday life that are normal to you can be painful for me.	7.	Be patient and consistent; I learn better when you tell, show and do things with me.
3.	It isn't that I don't listen to you... it's just that I can't understand you.	8.	Focus and build on what I can do rather than what I can't do.
4.	I like routines because I know what to expect.	9.	I want to be with others but I don't know how.
5.	Don't compare me with other children... I am special in my own way.	10.	Love me unconditionally, because I promise you I am worth it.

http://www.RaisingAutisticKids.com, (2015)

Chapter 2

The Child's Perspective

Developmentally Appropriate Practice

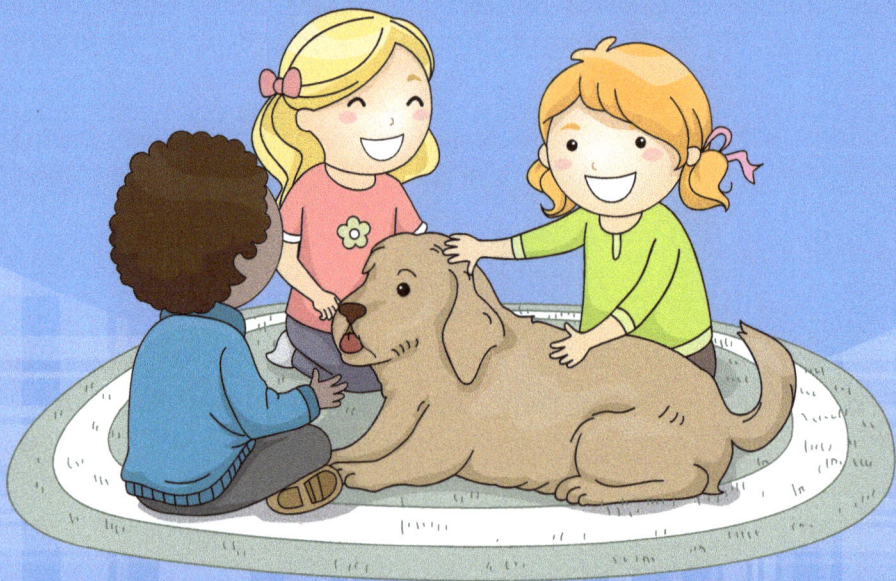

The Child-centered Classroom: Meeting the Needs of All

Before we can begin to discuss working with children with special needs, it's important to take some time to look at the needs of young children in general. Sometimes teachers, with the best of intentions, are anxious to focus solely on the needs of two or three children in the classroom- especially if those little ones are demonstrating behavior issues. Actually, before focusing on those students, we need to take a look at the strategies and supports that are in place for the entire class. These tips, strategies and supports are helpful for all children, and set a tone of mutual respect, **predictability** and positive relationships. Think of these as the foundation you are building upon in your classroom. We have to know and address what helps typical children achieve success because meeting those needs may well make a huge positive difference for many of your students with special needs as well. It's just good teaching; it's no biggie!

Consider the young child's perspective. Pretend for a moment that you are a four-year-old preschooler attending a child care center for the first time. Up until now, you have always been in the care of friends or family. These people know your likes and dislikes and are anxious to make you happy. They are dedicated to meeting your needs all of the time by playing with you, talking with you, giving you individual attention. Lucky you! Suddenly, you are put into a situation where you are sharing one adult with ten or twelve other kids, all of whom have just as many needs as you do. You are sharing adult time and attention for the first time ever. These kids may demonstrate different social skills, throw tantrums, shout out, get physical with you during play, take things away from you or ignore you. The classroom may be loud, bright and crowded; the teacher may not pay much attention to you or to your needs, either physically or emotionally. This teacher will tell you when to eat, what to eat, what to play with and with whom to play. You are told when to go to the bathroom, when to go outside, when to be social and when to be quiet. You can't leave! You are stuck in this same room, with these same people and these same toys day after day after day. Would the four-year-old you want *you* for a teacher?

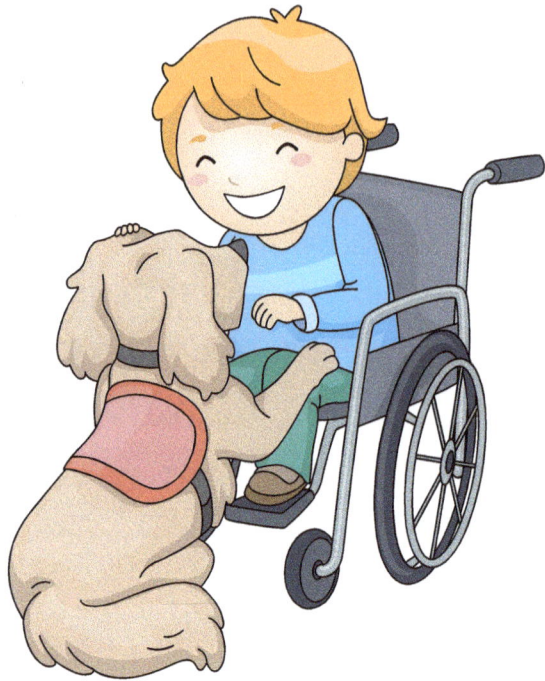

As an adult, how would you feel if you had to work in an office all day every day that you found too crowded, too stressful and you were doing a job that left you frustrated and angry every day when you went home? Perhaps your boss tells you that you may not leave the room until 5:00, tells you what you are having for lunch (whether it's something you like or not) tells you when you can go to the bathroom, who you must sit by and gives you no choice or say in the day's activities. You don't really enjoy your coworkers or your apathetic supervisor, but you are stuck with them in very close quarters anyway. Chances are, you would probably be looking for a different job that allowed you more flexibility and autonomy. You would look for a job that would allow you to feel valued, where your unique characteristics are appreciated and celebrated. That's what an adult would choose to do to; he would leave a situation that wasn't working for him.

We must recognize that young children don't have that option. Our little ones are totally dependent on us to make their days enjoyable and their time with us valuable, no matter what their abilities. As teachers, we have a moral and ethical obligation to provide the best possible experience for all the children in our care, and to meet their individual needs. Even in the highest quality setting, meeting all the needs of all of your little ones is an ongoing challenge.

Some children love the busy, active child care setting and thrive there. For others, including many children on the autism spectrum, the situation is stressful and unpleasant. Many little ones will struggle to keep up with daily activities while others will need more challenge and stimulation than what the typical classroom provides. Some students will need accommodations and extra help from you in making the experience successful. Others will challenge you to think differently and to expand your knowledge and skills set. A good teacher can match the environment, expectations and relationships to the needs of individual children and not to treat the classroom as a "one size fits all" factory. Adhering to good developmentally appropriate practices, being good observers and building positive relationships will go a long way in meeting the needs of your little ones. Sometimes a teacher is concerned about a child's development and may even want a child evaluated for special education, when really just focusing on best practice will remedy the concerns. Special education may not be needed. Teachers must first understand typical child development and educational principles before they can understand children with special needs.

Children don't have adult brains. Their problem solving abilities and coping skills are limited, even in the best of circumstances. Children by nature are egocentric and are not able to see your perspective on things. A child on the spectrum certainly won't see things from your point of view. That's why it is so important that those of us who work with young children always keep the child's perspective in mind. Just like adults, each child has different needs, preferences and limits, gifts and talents. Get to know your children well and develop personal relationships with each child. Know what rewards Daniel or upsets Tim. Know what strategies help Tina with her delayed language development and how to meet Justin's sensory needs. These are some of the tools in the teacher bag of tricks that make the difference between a teacher who runs a factory and a great teacher who is there to make a positive difference in the lives all children, including those with autism and other special needs.

Take a minute or two occasionally to think about how your classroom would feel to a new child coming in for the first time. Is it welcoming and pleasant? Is it a cheerful place to spend time? Is it too loud, too bright, too crowded, or too dim? What are your interactions with the children like? How do you feel about spending time in your classroom? If you don't love it there yourself, maybe it's time to make some positive changes.

🔑 KEY POINTS

- Children's problem solving skills and coping skills are limited. They depend on us for guidance.
- Before looking at specific child behaviors, examine your classroom environment as a whole.
- The better you know each child individually, the better you will be able to respond to their needs.
- If you don't love being in your classroom, make some positive changes.
- Always keep the child's perspective in mind.

The Physical Environment

We know it is always easier to prevent problems by being proactive than to respond after the fact, or to be re-active. The way you look at the physical environment in your classroom can help you create a positive, proactive learning situation that meets the needs of all children.

The physical environment of a classroom can affect behaviors and attitudes of both children and adults. Your goal is to set up your classroom space in such a way that it meets the needs of the children in your care. Take a look around your classroom from the child's perspective. If a classroom has every inch of the wall covered with posters and pictures, it may be visually overwhelming for some children. Have you ever been in a room that was so "busy" you couldn't wait to get out of it? Some teachers seem to think that every poster they have ever purchased over their entire teaching career should be displayed in the classroom at all times. After a very short time in that room, a child could find himself so visually overwhelmed that he may act out. We fill our classrooms with beautiful and wonderful things and then spend our days frustrated because the children won't pay attention to us. They prefer to look around at the classroom full of glorious and enchanting things, and then get in trouble for it!

If your room is too "busy," limit the items you put up on the wall. If you have shelves full of interesting items, you may want to reduce the visual stimulation by simply covering some of the shelves with a plain colored sheet. You can make a custom curtain for the front of your shelves with the help of a sewing machine, or a teacher's best friend, Velcro™.

On the other hand, is your room too bare and sparse? The children in your care are often spending more awake time in that classroom during the week than they are at home. Does your room look engaging, welcoming, and friendly? Do the wall colors and carpets invite children to come in or turn them away? What about lighting? If the overhead lighting is too harsh, consider some lamps or other alternatives. Do you have windows? Are you making the most of a beautiful view, if you are lucky enough to have one? Are you maximizing the amount of light that can be allowed into the room? Have you considered some type of window covering, shade, or curtains that are appealing to the eye? Doing all you can to make your space appealing and comfortable is well worth the payback you get in improved behaviors and positive attitudes- in both adults and children. Garage sales, dollar stores, putting the word out through social media and letting your classroom parents know about your needs can all help you find items to make your environment more comfortable for all.

Need ideas? A web search for images of "high quality preschool environments" will give you more great ideas than you will need in this lifetime. A Pinterest.com search will yield great results as well.

Part of your job as a teacher is to structure the physical environment for success. The environment clearly tells what your expectations are as far as caring for materials and putting things away. Photos can be a great tool to let kids know exactly what you expect of them. Many children don't comply because they really don't know what's expected of them. Children on the autism spectrum or with developmental delays will appreciate added visual support. Be creative in thinking about how you can use visuals to support your classroom expectations. Your camera is your best friend in the classroom!

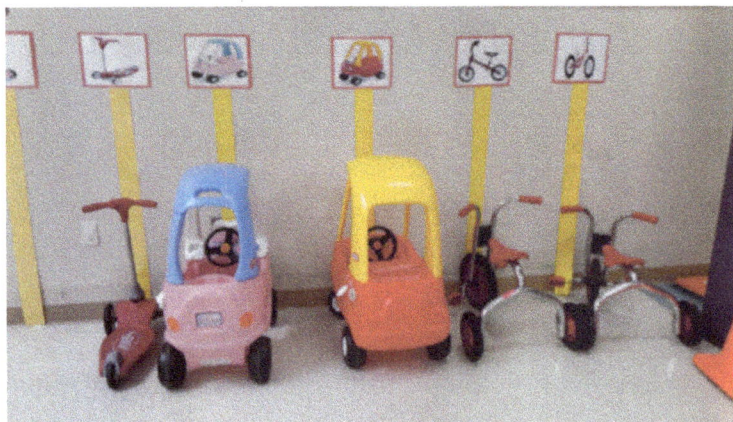

Here is a good functional example for parking the bikes at the end of an indoor play session. Simple reminders can be posted in the physical environment to provide consistency for everyone, as well as providing verbal cues and common language that adults can use consistently.

Often squabbles arise over toys and materials. Do you have enough engaging, interesting toys and items in the classroom for the

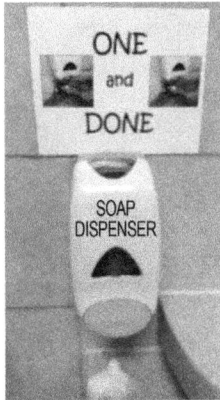

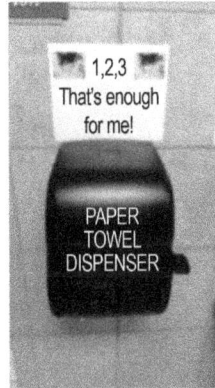

number of children you have in your care? Broken toys, tattered books and puzzles with missing pieces don't count. A visiting teacher once sat down with a child in a classroom to do a puzzle together. They dumped out the large box of puzzle pieces, and within a few minutes the teacher began to wonder what good that master's degree had really done her. Neither the teacher nor the child could get any pieces to fit. Then, the five-year-old child and teacher figured out that there were actually four different puzzles all dumped together in that one box. Talk about frustrating! The classroom teacher wondered why no students ever played with that box of puzzles. Have a variety of interesting, engaging, age-appropriate toys and materials to keep your class busy and happy.

Be respectful of kids when you ask them to share. Nobody wants to turn over a project he has been working on for 30 minutes to someone else, and let that new person take over, whether it is a child or an adult. Some materials lend themselves better to turn taking rather than sharing, and that's okay. A turn taking sign up sheet that the children can see might help prevent problems, teach turn taking, and provide a literacy opportunity as well.

Kids need variety. Change out center materials when interest begins to wane. Children love open ended materials that help them create and problem solve. A variety of sizes of boxes for building, a couple sets of measuring cups for water play, scraps of wrapping paper to cut up are all conducive to creative fun. These are the simple things that can make a child's day. Take a look around the room weekly to see what materials need to be discarded, repaired or changed out. If a toy hasn't been played with for a couple of weeks, give it a rest and bring it out again in a few weeks for a novel experience. Sometimes just changing the color of the Play-Doh® or adding a few things to the housekeeping center makes a big difference and will prevent behavior issues that arise from children who are bored. Be sure that your toys and materials are not too easy (boring) or too difficult (frustrating) for the majority of the children in your classroom.

What is the traffic flow pattern in your classroom? If everybody needs to walk right through the block center to get to the bathroom and it's creating problems for the block builders, you may need to change your classroom arrangement. Children should be able to have play spaces that are not highways. Small areas for play can be made by utilizing low shelves, seating, area rugs and other physical markers that designate specific areas for play and are out of the general traffic flow. Group noisier centers like blocks and housekeeping together and quieter centers such as the bookshelf, office/writing area or fine motor center closer together to help children follow through with your behavior expectations.

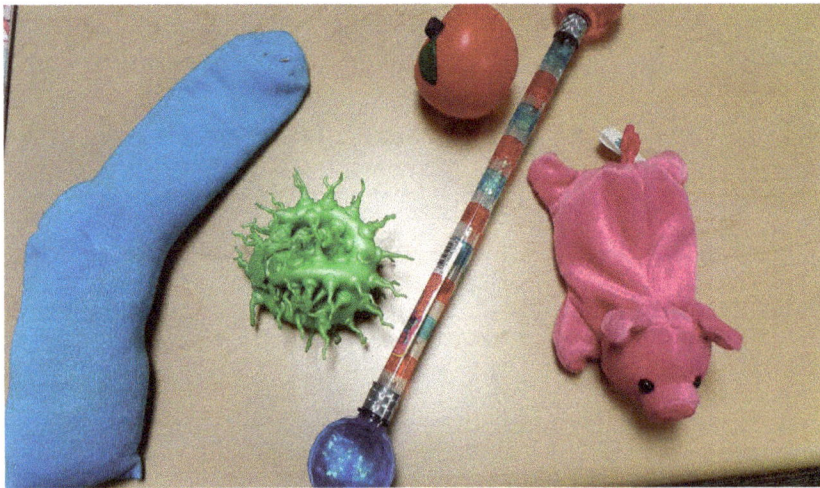

No matter how tiny your classroom space, allow a quiet area where a child can go to step out of the fray for a little while. This space is not a "time out" or punishment area but a place a child can choose to go to take a break, to relax with a stuffed animal or book, and take a deep breath before rejoining the group. A sensory bottle filled with oil, water and glitter can give the child something calming to land look at as he self-calms. This can be a lifesaver for a child with autism or sensory needs, and can really help those who become overwhelmed in the classroom environment. All of these things may help you prevent problems before they arise.

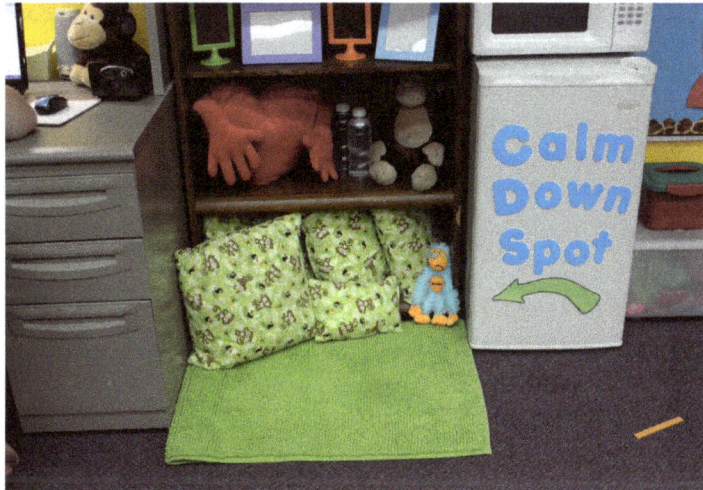

Image by Lisa Mongold, Preschool Teacher, Merrillville, Indiana.
https://lisamongold.wordpress.com

🔑 KEY POINTS

- Have well-defined areas for both active and quiet play.
- Provide toys that are appropriate for the age and developmental levels of the children.
- Provide enough toys and materials that children don't have to wait too long for turns or share toys that really don't lend themselves to sharing.
- Change up materials frequently to keep interest levels high.

The Social-Emotional Environment

Research has proven time and time again that the variable that makes the most difference in any classroom is a caring teacher. Your attitude toward and your relationship with your students has far more effect than a fancy playground or expensive toys ever could. The quality of the relationship you have with your students defines the quality of care they receive on a daily basis. We often find ourselves as teachers getting frustrated with children's behavior, when maybe the first thing we should do is take a look at ourselves as teachers, and see what we can change first about our own behaviors and expectations.

Looking at things from a child's perspective, would *you* want to be a student in your classroom? Chances are, your four-year-old self would want a teacher who is kind, thoughtful, patient, caring, and provides a high degree of emotional safety.

We know that children are going to make mistakes. They don't have adult brains yet to help them to reason, plan ahead, see the consequences of their actions and to solve problems. Children need adults in their lives who understand that, and are willing to help them learn social skills and problem solving skills in a kind, gentle way, not through humiliation and punishment. We don't expect children to come to school knowing how to read and write, but somehow we do often expect them to come with an adult set of social skills. If that is your expectation as a teacher, you will continually be disappointed in your little ones as they have much learning and growing to do in that area. If you understand that, you have the amazing opportunity to help these children learn problem solving and social skills on a daily basis. They are learning from your example every minute. Children with autism will especially need you to be a consistent presence in their lives, one they can count on for support and guidance in navigating their preschool world.

While all children have a need for routine and consistency in their day, this is especially true for those on the spectrum. Think about the last time you went to an inservice, a board meeting, or even a wedding. The first thing you look for is some sort of a program or agenda. You want to know how long you will be at this event, and what you will be doing while you are there. Children like to know what to expect when they are at school.

Sometimes teachers post classroom rules (that the kids can't read), and think that covers all the bases, but that only works if the students are aware of the rules and why they are in place.

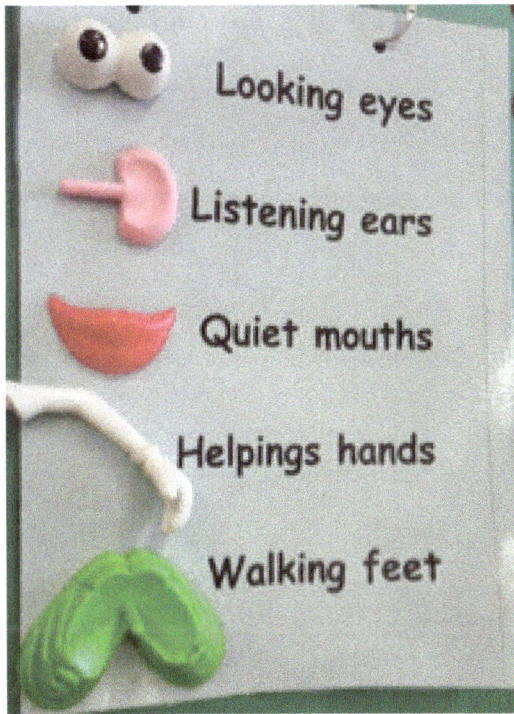

Looking eyes

Listening ears

Quiet mouths

Helpings hands

Walking feet

Your students can help you brainstorm important rules for the classroom; and remember, less is better when it comes to rules. The more the students are involved in determining the rules, and the more child-friendly the language, the more they will buy into them.

With your students, repetition is key. Rules need to be talked about and reinforced daily in appropriate, meaningful ways to be effective.

Establishing relationships with your students is a fundamental building block for learning. A therapist visited a school on a weekly basis. Every time she was there, she could hear the teacher in the next room yelling at her class. Every week she heard the same verbal assault coming from the room next door. The student the therapist was working with often commented, "That teacher is yelling." After 30 minutes of this, both therapist and student could feel their anxiety levels go up. Imagine being a little three-year-old child in that classroom. That teacher was not only failing to develop a positive relationship with her students, she was actively guaranteeing their relationship would be a negative one. Luckily for all, that teacher was replaced early in the semester.

There are two little checkpoints to use in building your relationships with children. First, ask yourself if you would you speak the same way to the child if his parent were standing right behind you. Monitor both your words and your tone. Even very young children or those on the autism spectrum will notice your tone, whether they understand your words or not. Secondly, picture these little people all grown up and talking about their memories of you as a preschool teacher. They may not remember all the activities you did, the songs you sang or the artwork they created, but they will remember how you made them feel. Your students are tiny people now that will grow into adults later, and the way you treat them will leave a mark on their lives. What memories will they have of you, and of how you treated them? When they grow up to be parents, teachers, attorneys, ball players and mechanics later in life, what will they remember about you? Is your tone of voice kind and calm or loud and abusive? Are you working to build relationships with these small people in your care, or are you using your position simply to gain power and control over them?

Be sure to establish some rituals in your classroom to help develop a sense of community among your students. Have some songs, games, and routines that you do daily that recognize your children individually in fun, respectful, positive ways. Everybody needs to feel like he belongs. Everyone wants to be noticed and validated.

One way to show respect for children is to get down on their level when you speak to them. Use a calm, controlled voice and do not yell at them from across the room. Yelling will surely escalate the situation, will create more stress, and is ineffective in the long term. Walk over to the child to speak with him. Show him the same respect you would any friend. A child learns what respect looks like when you model it for him. Never forget that you are there to meet the needs of the child. He is not there to meet yours!

Give your students every opportunity to be actively involved in classroom decisions and plans. Ask them to help you make the little decisions. Consider their opinion as to what you should put in the block area that would be fun, or where you should we put a pretty new plant. When you do this, you meet the child's need for belonging and for some power and control. You are telling them that you respect them and value them enough to want their input.

Set reasonable limits and enforce them consistently. Be certain your students know exactly what your expectations are, and don't change your expectations from day to day. For example,

"Time to pick up blocks," seems pretty simple. However, that may convey a different meaning to two different people. To one, it may mean putting all the blocks in the giant block box, or putting them anywhere on the block shelf. To another person, it might mean that every block is put away in a specific place, according to shape. Expectations for even the simplest of tasks must be clearly demonstrated. Students on the spectrum will especially appreciate your consistency.

Model problem solving skills for your little ones. Children learn how to respond to difficult situations by watching how the adults in the environment handle those situations. A teaching assistant dropped an entire plastic pitcher of red juice (when kids still drank red juice at school) on a table full of children. The pitcher hit the table, bounced, and sprayed juice everywhere. The room looked like a crime scene. The adults in the room made a concerted effort to laugh about the whole incident with the kids as everyone got involved in the cleanup process with wet wipes and towels. Although it was a horrible mess, the teachers concentrated primarily on modeling problem solving skills with the kids and helping them to feel competent by being involved in the cleanup process. Everybody went home a little sticky, but it made a great story for the kids to tell, and wasn't worth anger. Some of the students who frustrate you the most are probably the ones who are not able to problem solve effectively. This will include your students with autism and developmental delays.

Real, true self-esteem comes from acquiring competence. Children don't develop self-esteem because someone is continually telling them how wonderful they are. Self-esteem comes from feeling competent in handling the everyday problems and frustrations in life. Do not rob your children of the opportunity to develop those skills. Let them learn to handle small problems, whatever their ability level, so that they can gradually learn to handle bigger problems as they grow older.

🔑 KEY POINTS

- Treat your students with respect and kindness. They are people who just happen to be smaller than you. Developing positive relationships matter more than anything else you do.
- Set reasonable limits and enforce them consistently.
- Involve children in the decision making process whenever appropriate.
- Model problem solving.
- Self-esteem comes from acquiring competence. Teachers assist children in learning to be competent in everyday life.

Teaching **transitions** is an effective way to help children learn competence in their everyday environment. So often, when students have difficulties managing themselves, it's at transition times. This may be when they are going outside, down the hall to lunch, leaving circle time for centers, etc. Times like these give you the opportunity to practice being a creative problem solver. If you are sending too many kids to the same place at the same time, you will have problems. Find a way to send them in a little slower, more measured way. For example, announce that everybody wearing blue, or everybody wearing socks, or if your name starts with the letter J may go next. In addition to helping maintain order in the transition, you are turning the activity itself into a teachable moment. Have some quick, easy songs or rhymes in your teacher bag of tricks that you can call upon to help children recognize transitions and what you expect of them at that time. One sign of a good teacher is the ability to move a group of children from one activity to another in a fun, engaging, positive way.

Be ready to assist with the transition by moving yourself as the majority of the group moves. Be proactive in spotting problems and helping those who need your assistance during the transition. Children thrive on routine and will respond well to a predictable song at cleanup time. One class tried to get the room picked up before the three-minute song ended, and loved that daily game. As you're cleaning up, children loved to be told, "you are in charge of the block area today," or "you are the book boss, please make sure all the books go back on the shelf." Expect that these children are young, and they will be easily overwhelmed by trying to do too much (just as you are with too much housework on a day off) and multiple directions. It's always a good idea to give a five-minute warning, especially to those who are really engaged, or in their favorite center. Teach your specific expectations- otherwise, how do your students know what you expect? A good teacher has a bag of transition tricks to draw from, anticipates that these are the times when problems will occur and is ready to help the little ones work through this learning.

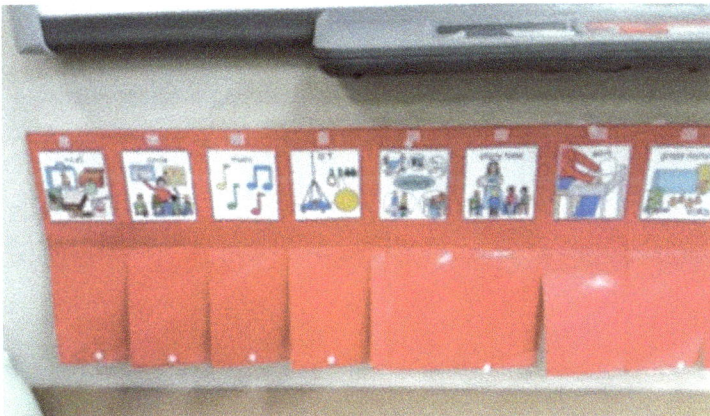

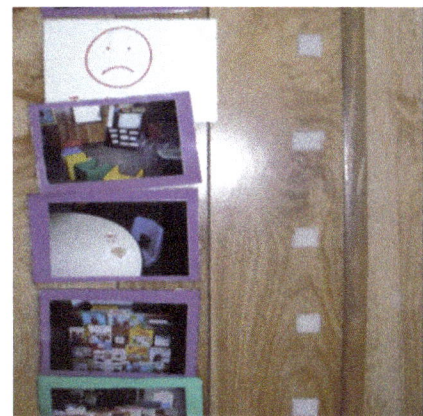

If you don't already use some sort of a class picture schedule in your room, start doing it. That will help all of your students know what to anticipate, what's next and will serve as their version of a day planner. This will especially help students with autism, cognitive and language delays. An online search for "picture schedule" or "visual class schedule" will give you a myriad of ideas. Just like any strategy, model how it works for your students and use it daily. Make it a part of your daily routine, and you will see your students refer to it for information. These pages have a few examples.

The sad face on the vertical schedule indicates that this will be an inside day due to weather, no playground. It is switched out with a playground picture and a question mark for the days that a decision about outside time can't be made until later in the day. You can change the pictures when needed for schedule changes. Stock photos can be found, but children love to see themselves in their very own classroom doing what they do, so you may want to take your own photos for the schedule.

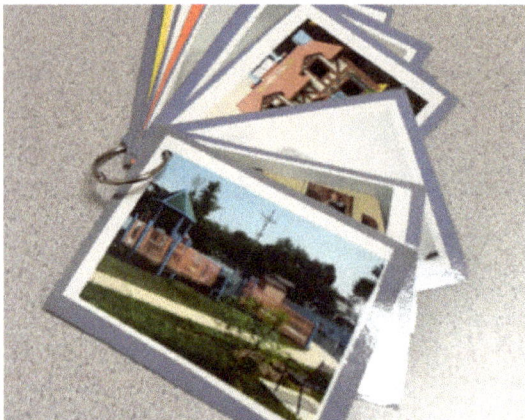

A set of pictures on a ring can go with you to the playground, lunchroom or library. These visuals can serve as a reminder about about the next activity. For some students that have trouble transitioning, a portable "schedule" like this can be comforting.

A student who needs a schedule that is more individualized and specific to their day may benefit from something tailored to their needs.

Another helpful class-wide strategy is a visual timer. This can help the entire class see how much time is left in an activity, such as center time. It can be used specifically for an individual student who has trouble with transitions or staying on task. Timers remove the burden from the teacher. For example, the timer says it's time to pick up, rather than the teacher making this demand. The timer says it's time to come in from outside play, rather than the teacher having to be "responsible" for that unpopular decision. It seems a small point, but can really make a noticeable difference. These are available online and at teacher supply stores.

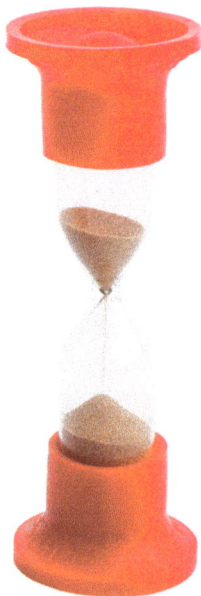

🔑 KEY POINTS

- A picture is worth a thousand words.
- A visual support may be a picture or a tangible object.
- Visual supports can help with transitions.
- Teaching children to transition from one activity to the next is helpful to them as well as to the teacher.
- Visual timers are a wonderful tool to help children acquire a sense of time and transition.
- Use of visual schedules is a way to give children knowledge of what comes next.
- Visual schedules using pictures of the children themselves is especially effective.

When you encounter behavior issues, often the best option with very young children is simply to redirect them to another activity. Little ones are not making bad choices just to make you angry. They are in the process of learning expectations and problem solving. As children reach the age of four or five, it's important for the teacher to understand the difference between punishment and discipline. Sometimes those terms are used interchangeably, and they really mean different things.

Punishment is defined as a punitive correction for misbehavior. In other words, "You did something wrong, and you must pay." Often the punishment does not relate directly to the offense, and thereby loses effectiveness. For example, a child who misbehaves may be punished by missing outdoor time, a class party, or by being made to write "I will not kick the dog" one hundred times.

Discipline (comes from the word "disciple": someone who learns) is thought of in the early childhood world as teaching; we teach positive alternatives, talk with the child about what could be done differently next time, and support children as they make those changes. We help the child recognize and deal with strong emotions, and work through the situation. Those mistakes are recognized as learning opportunities, and the teacher recognizes that skills of any sort are only learned through practice. Discipline involves being engaged with the child and teaching them what you want them to do. So many of our children misbehave because they have not been taught what behaviors are expected of them. Take for example a child who has a tantrum and throws a handful of Legos© against the wall. Discipline might be characterized by waiting until the child calms down (because it is pointless to try to reason with an angry or out of control child) then working with him to pick up the Legos©. At that point give the child ideas about what he can do next time he is angry or frustrated when the Legos© refuse to cooperate in building exactly what the child wants. In *Tic Toc Autism Clock: A Guide to Your 24/7 Plan*, Barboa and Obrey (2015) describe this as a ChoicesChat©. [5]

Bijou, Peterson and Ault (1968) developed a system of behavior management they called **Anecdotal Observation**, known as **ABC Recording**. [6] This system looks at the **antecedent** (what happened right before the behavior occurred) the **behavior** itself, and the **consequence** of the behavior (what happened right after the behavior). Using this simple system can help you be a behavior detective and figure out why things might be happening the way they are.

BEHAVIOR TRACKING CHART

Date/Time	Activity	Antecedent	Behavior	Consequence
Date/Time when behavior occurred	What activity was going on when the behavior occurred; who was present?	What happened right before the behavior that may have triggered the behavior?	What did the behavior look like, what was the duration and intensity?	What happened after the behavior, or as a result of the behavior?

The ABC method of charting follows a simple formula. Remove the emotions, just examine the facts and this technique will lead you to the answers you are seeking.

A. What is the *antecedent*, (the thing that happens right before the behavior occurs)? This could be a specific directive, the involvement of a specific person, a specific place or situation.

 B. What is the *behavior* you are seeing? How long does the behavior last, how intense is it, and how often does it occur?

C. What is the *consequence* of the behavior? Is the child getting something he wants, or is he avoiding something he doesn't want? For behaviors to continue, there has to be some sort of payoff for the child. Think of the "consequence" from the child's perspective. Some teachers impose a consequence they think will eliminate the behavior when in reality it only serves to increase it.

 Like most children, William enjoys individualized attention from the teacher. When there is a large group activity in the classroom, William acts out loudly, disturbing the others and preventing them from learning. One of the teachers removes him from the group and sits with him individually and reads to him to settle him down. He is training her well to get exactly what he wants from her- individual attention. She is totally reinforcing the unwanted behavior. When you use the ABC recording chart to document behavior concerns, you might see that those children who are *sensory avoiding* may try to escape activities that are far too stimulating, or overfill their cups. [6]

 Ethan was a five-year-old boy, who was extremely sensitive to too much noise and activity in his environment. When Ethan, a very bright boy, went from a home child care setting to a child care center, it was very traumatic for him. The child care center was noisy and chaotic. Ethan tried to find ways to avoid the sensory overload by going to a corner of the room or not lining up right away with everyone else. He found the presence of children so close to him and putting hands all over him to be very upsetting. His avoidance behaviors would result in him getting in trouble with the teacher. She would get in his face, get loud, and then get more upset when Ethan tried to run away from her. [8]

A quick use of the ABC behavior chart, and doing some objective observations over a period of a few days helped the teacher to see that Ethan was only trying to avoid situations he found overwhelming. In addition, the teacher became more aware of her own behavior, and found that working with Ethan using a team approach was a much better solution. She was able to have a good, long conversation with Ethan about some of the things he found upsetting in the classroom, and they reached some compromises. She allowed Ethan to be last in line to allow him the option of giving himself some additional space with his peers. He was allowed to sit at the very edge of the group at circle time. He was provided a quiet space in a corner of the classroom to go to, *not* as a time out, but as a place he could go when the room overwhelmed him.

As a result, the teacher began to look at Ethan in a different light. Instead of dwelling on her concerns about him, she began to focus on his strengths. The teacher started to allow Ethan the opportunity to help in the classroom and around the school in informal ways. This seemed to help to give him a sense of having some power each day, and to increase adult interactions, which the teacher had observed he really enjoyed. In a week, Ethan's problem behaviors had diminished by nearly 90%, and everyone was much happier. Ethan's initial misbehavior in the classroom was communicating that the environment was far too sensory rich for him. He just needed the teacher to realize that his behavior *was* communication.

Other positive discipline strategies might include developing reasonable classroom limits to prevent behaviors before they occur, teaching problem solving skills, and being proactive (rather than re-active). Give guidance to children you notice having trouble, using diverting and distracting techniques. Offer positive choices, and help children preserve their dignity in a discipline encounter (not yelling at a child across a room, but rather having a private conversation). Be supportive of a child in a discipline encounter rather than being angry. Have you ever been disciplined in front of all of your peers? Ouch! We wouldn't yell at a child who was struggling with learning to count, so why would we yell at a child who is struggling to learn social behaviors?

Finally, are you having fun every day in your classroom? Are your kids having fun every day? You should all be having fun! Be a little silly, laugh a lot, hug, chat and create! The opportunity to spend time with children is an amazing gift. Be sure every day is joyful, energizing and meaningful. You will be surprised at the difference your positive attitude makes.

KEY POINTS

- Children's problem solving skills and coping skills are limited. They depend on adults to help handle difficult situations.
- The single most important thing you can do with your students is to build positive relationships in your classroom.
- Your classroom should be a happy place to be for both children and adults; kids will remember how you made them feel.
- Set reasonable limits and enforce them consistently and kindly.
- Teach children the specific skills they need to meet your expectations.
- Be proactive rather than re-active to discipline problems. Anticipate when and where problems are most likely to occur and head them off.

The Cognitive/Learning Environment

Sometimes teachers get frustrated with a child's behavior when actually there is not a good fit between the teaching that is happening in the classroom and a child's developmental level or learning needs. In early childhood, we talk about **developmentally appropriate practice**, or teaching in a way that meets the developmental needs of our students. This means understanding what children are able to do at different ages and stages of development, and keeping the learning meaningful and relevant to that particular stage. A good teacher knows not to expect more than a child is capable of learning. A good reminder is, "You can't teach a child to develop," and that is so true.

Think about child development in terms of learning to ride a bicycle. Almost every child will eventually learn to ride a bike. However, we would not expect a two-year-old child to have mastered the complex set of cognitive and motor skills that is necessary for that physical feat. Pushing and prodding, repeated practice, rewards and praise have no effect if a child is simply not ready to master the skill. In fact, pushing a skill too early can actually be detrimental. The child is not ready to ride the bike, gets hurt (physically and emotionally) and then decides not to ever try to ride a bike again. We would never, in good conscience, push a child to master a physical skill like bike riding, jumping rope, skateboarding, even going up and down stairs, until he has the ability to do it. However, sometimes we forget and expect more in terms of pre-academics than a child is ready for, and that can do real damage.

As teachers, focus on skills that fall within the child's **zone of proximal development (ZPD)**. [7] This refers to the skills that fall somewhere between what a child is unable to do, and what he can do completely independently. The ZPD is the magic zone where we can "scaffold" the child's learning to independence. This concept was popularized by Soviet psychologist Lev Vygotsky. [7] To do this effectively, it is vital that a teacher knows and understands what typical development looks like to help the child reach the very next level.

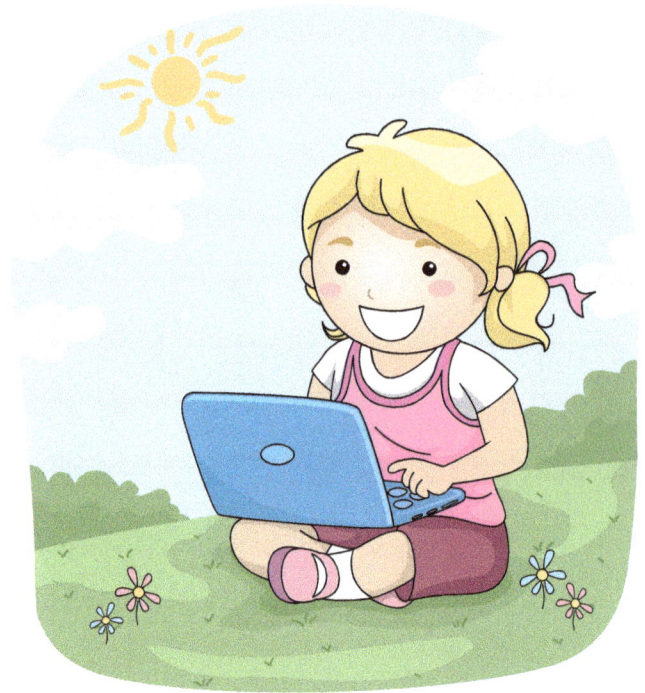

Children with autism may have acquired skills and abilities that are out of developmental sequence. Some skills may be very low, some right on track and some really advanced. This is why it is so important to know your children individually. You cannot fully understand "atypical" children until you know what's typical. Look online to discover websites you can access for reliable developmental charts detailing typical childhood milestones. Your special needs students may not follow these norms, but you need to know what is typical development for most children in order to step outside the developmental box and create meaningful learning for those who don't fit the mold.

How do children learn best? The research is exceedingly clear on this. Young children are meant to be active beings. Children learn through using all their senses, moving their whole bodies and being engaged with hands-on activities that challenge them to think creatively and explore their environment naturally. This means providing real life materials, toys that engage the creative brain and allowing movement in your classroom.

Worksheets are not the way young children learn. A child may be able to "complete" a worksheet, but that doesn't mean he has learned the concept. In addition, many of the color, cut and paste activity sheets simply ask more of a child's organizational skills than their developmental capabilities allow. Think of a worksheet showing a picture of a house with the typical directions, "Color it, cut it out, do your best work. Color in the lines. Stay in your seat until you are finished."

Compare this to an activity in which children are encouraged to build houses for some teddy bears. In this activity the children are given a variety of materials: cardboard scraps, fabric, colored paper, pipe cleaners, plastic cups, wooden blocks, scissors, and glue. They are told to work with their neighbor to build a house. Picture how that classroom looks. In coloring a house, you will see children sitting in their chairs, working quietly.

In the second activity, you will see children practicing language and problem solving skills, learning about simple physics, sharing, cooperating and moving around the center as they work. The second scenario takes more preparation on the part of the teacher. The finished product may not be as "slick" looking, but the children are learning far more by engaging in a hands-on learning activity.

With worksheet-type activities, you will always have a portion of the children in your classroom who find this activity too difficult, and others who find it too easy and are bored (so you are not teaching in the zone of proximal development for these children, right?) [7]

With open-ended activities, you, as a teacher, will have a far better idea of your children's capabilities. This is especially important in working with children with special needs because we sometimes have pre-conceived ideas of what they should and should not be able to do, and we are often wrong about that.

A story that illustrates this perfectly involved Karen, who was identified as being on the autism spectrum. The special education teacher visited Karen's preschool classroom briefly each week, and her job was to help Karen with her work which was typically a worksheet or a teacher directed activity. One day, the activity consisted of putting a sticker skeleton together on a piece of paper; the teacher was then handing the students a sticker with the corresponding name of the bone and telling them where to put it. Karen was handed the sticker with the word "knee." She told her special helper that must be the wrong word, since it began with a k, but quickly self- corrected, and told her that it must be a silent k. Upon a little further investigation, the visiting teacher found that Karen was reading a number of words. When this was mentioned to her classroom teacher, she had no idea that Karen had this skill. Every activity in that classroom was so teacher directed that she had no idea many of her students were able to go far beyond the worksheets they were asked to do in class, including Karen. Open-ended activities allow you to observe not only the students who are able to go farther and challenge themselves, but also those students who are struggling with more basic concepts and may need more of your assistance to move forward at their own pace. Children on the autism spectrum may have skills that surprise you, and that you may never see demonstrated unless you allow them the opportunity.

For preschoolers, learning is about the process, not the finished product. Sometimes we, as adults, get so wrapped up in what something should look like, we forget that it's the process that is far more important.

When we talk about "play" and children, remember that play is an activity that is freely chosen by the child. If you are directing the child to spend time in a center not of his choosing for either more or less time than he wants, that becomes work and not play.

There is nothing wrong with having some directed activities during the day, especially in small groups, but your day must contain plenty of time for hands-on, active learning. This allows you to meet the needs of all your students, regardless of their learning level, and to structure the activities to meet each student's learning style.

🔑 KEY POINTS

- Research clearly indicates that children learn best through hands-on, active play. Allowing for learning through play will prevent many behavior issues.
- Teach to the child's zone of proximal development. [7]
- Real learning for young children is about the process, not the finished product.
- Sometimes both teacher and child are frustrated when there is not a good match between the way the teacher structures learning in the classroom and the way the child actually learns.
- Open-ended activities will help you learn much about your little one's capabilities.

Chapter 3

The Parents' Perspective

Realities and Responsibilities

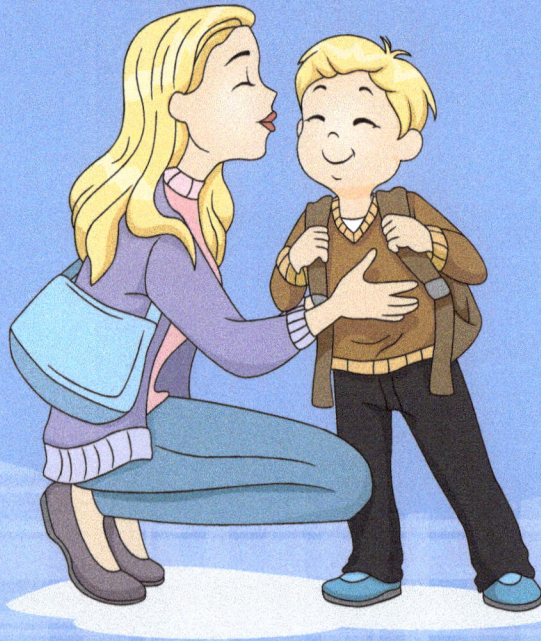

Working with young children necessitates working with their parents.

This is especially true of children who may have some learning differences or challenging behaviors. You may encounter parents who have been living with an autism or other diagnosis for their child for several years. They may be well on the road to acceptance. On the other hand, you may have a child in your classroom with a diagnosis that is very new and painful for the family. You may encounter parents who have not begun the diagnostic process or even consulted with a physician about their concerns regarding their child's development. All families you serve will work with their child in a little different way. Much depends on how intimidating the thought of raising a child with special needs is to that particular family. You see the child in the fairly isolated context of your own classroom, so you may be seeing only the tip of the iceberg of concerns the parents are facing.

Here are some of the questions and challenges that parents may be thinking about on a daily basis:

- Is there really anything "wrong" with my child? Should we get a second or even third opinion?
- Two different doctors are telling us two different things. To whom should we listen?
- How do we share this information with grandparents, aunts, and uncles? Should we say anything? Will they notice?
- How will this affect our other children? Will they have to give up activities just so we can pay for therapy? Will they resent their sibling for the time and energy he takes?
- Different agencies offer different therapies. Which are right for our child?
- What will this do to our adult relationship/marriage?
- How will we pay for all these recommended therapies?   Are they really necessary?
- Will this child care center ask my child to leave just like the previous two did? Will they be able to meet his needs? Will they be kind to him even when he is having a hard day?
- Will they love him like we do?
- Will he ever be toilet trained? Will he ever have a job?

- What if something happens to us? Who will take care of him?
- How can I give this child the time and resources he needs while still taking care of my other children?
- What do people think of me and my family? Is everyone judging me?
- How can I get enough sleep to care for myself and the rest of my family with a child who stays up all night?
- How can I keep my home safe and keep him from running away or wandering off?

Work hard to be honest but kind as you share concerns with parents. Put yourself in their place and think about how your words sound. If you have a difficult conference or parent meeting coming up, don't hesitate to practice with a co-worker. Thinking through the various paths the conference may take can sometimes help you to think through what to say, and how to make the meeting less stressful. Always remind parents that you are on their side and that all of you want what is best for the child. The best communication is not aggressive, not passive, but is assertive, and tells the truth in a thoughtful and considerate way (NAEYC, 1998). [8]

Recognize that parents may be going through a grieving process as they mourn the ideal child they thought they would have and learn to work with the child they actually have, including the good and the difficult, the rewarding and the challenging. As much as the parents love this child, it takes a shift in thinking as they begin to process the idea of parenting a child with some special needs (Healey, 1996). [9] Parents may actually go through a grief process similar to that of a person who has lost a loved one to death. For some parents, a diagnosis *is* actually a   death of their dreams of the perfect child, the perfect family life, and the perfect future for that child. At first parents may be in shock, then denial that the problem actually exists, or that a diagnosis has been given. This stage may be followed by anger. At this point, the parent may rage at anyone who comes too "close" to acknowledgement of the diagnosis, and may verbally attack others such as teachers, therapists or child care providers, without thinking. It's important to understand as a teacher or child care provider that this is not about you. You may be the person the parent deals with most in connection with the child, and so you may be the one to bear the brunt of parental anger and frustration. Parents may look for something or someone, often including themselves, to blame for the diagnosis. "Is it because I had that one drink when I was seven months pregnant?" or "If only I had called the doctor sooner, we could have headed this off?" are examples of this type of thinking that is completely normal. Parents will eventually move to a point where they become resigned to the actuality of the diagnosis, and then are ready to move into the adjustment phase, as they work to create a new sort of life with new expectations.

As you work with parents, understand that this acceptance is a process that is a little bit different for everybody. Be patient as you work with parents because they are fighting a hard battle, and you may only see a tiny sliver of the issues they are facing. Teachers sometimes find that they have tremendous concerns about a student, try addressing it with the parents, and find that their voiced worries are met with anger or denial. Sometimes parents may need to hear concerns from a number of people in various places before they are actually able to begin the diagnostic process. Once it begins, it may give answers they are not yet ready to accept. Understand that this is a part of the diagnostic process.

As a teacher, your task is to be supportive of both parents and children, no matter where they may be on this journey. Sometimes a parent just needs a listening, non-judgmental ear, and you can fill that role. Other times a parent may come to you seeking advice or information about community resources and you are the person who serves as the link between the family and agencies or resources that can provide additional support. Do your professional homework and be ready to offer ideas of agencies that parents can contact for additional assistance. A good place to start when parents are ready to think about the testing process is your local school district. They will be able to provide assistance and testing for children as young as three, and can tell you what agency to call in your area that can provide services to children younger than three. The school district can also be a gateway to other services and agencies. Anytime you work with children and families, stay informed about what your community offers to families and who you can connect them with to get further information, but the school district is always a good place to start.

Try very hard to not only be the bearer of bad news, but the good also. All kids have challenges, but all kids have strengths as well. In teaching a child with social or learning concerns, it's easy to fall into the trap of focusing only on the deficit areas. Do yourselves and those over-stressed parents a favor and look for the positives also, because they are there. No parent wants to come pick their child up after a stressful day at work only to be met at the preschool door by an angry or frustrated teacher who is only too anxious to share with them all the things their child did wrong that day. Look for little signs of progress, and funny "typical" kid stories, along with any peer interactions you can note. Parents will be forever grateful to you for sharing some positives with them, and they will appreciate knowing that you are able to see the good in their child.

Understand what the parents are going through every day. Along with problems in sensory issues, social skills and communication, many children with autism face other medical challenges. A large number have seizures or sleep disorders. A teacher needs to be aware and prepared for the fact that the child (and indeed the whole family) may not have slept the night before and this can affect his classroom functioning. This goes on night after night for many families facing autism.

Many children with autism have **gastrointestinal issues** and require a special diet. You will need to maintain a child's diet diligently. Parents are trying to feed a healthy diet to children who, due to sensory or other issues, may be beyond picky. It is not at all unusual to find children on the spectrum who will only accept an extremely limited variety of foods.

Disorders that are affecting a child along with his autism are known as **concomitant disorders.** The number and severity of concomitant disorders that the child faces may be further complicated by medications he takes to remediate those other medical issues. Those pharmaceuticals may affect his classroom attention and behavior. Be very aware of all the health issues facing the children in your class and maintain close communication with the parent in relation to the child's health. If you work in a center that has access to medical services, such as a school nurse, establish a line of communication with the nurse regarding the child as soon as possible.

Allergies run rampant in this group of children, perhaps a function of their sensitivity to various stimuli. Be certain you are aware of what allergies (both food and environmental) each child has and be highly attentive to his possible exposure to the offending material. A child with an allergy to gluten may be so sensitive to it that he cannot even play with Play-Doh® types of compounds made with flour. A child with an allergy to banana may have a reaction from casually touching your hand after you held a banana. Dangerous nut allergies may be triggered by touching a counter top where nuts had previously been placed. Some lotions and other household items may contain the offending item, so get a detailed list from the parent and be certain that everyone at school follows the directives.

A common issue in children of this population is **attention deficit disorder** (ADD), sometimes combined with hyperactivity (ADHD). These issues, as well as other behavioral and medical diagnoses complicate the challenges of family life.

Having a child with special needs is draining on the family's emotions, time, and finances. Parents often sacrifice their own needs and well-being to give their children what is needed. They may be working an extra job to cover medical expenses. Understand that having a child on the spectrum totally changes the family dynamic and the demands faced by the family. Know that they need you, and you need to work closely with them.

KEY POINTS

- Children with ASD often have medical or behavioral issues that the parent must work with every day.
- Many children on the spectrum have dietary problems.
- A large number have environmental or food allergies that can be significant.
- Having a special needs child defines family life and requires a tremendous amount of time and family resources.

PART TWO
BEYOND THE BASICS

Chapter 4
Behavior

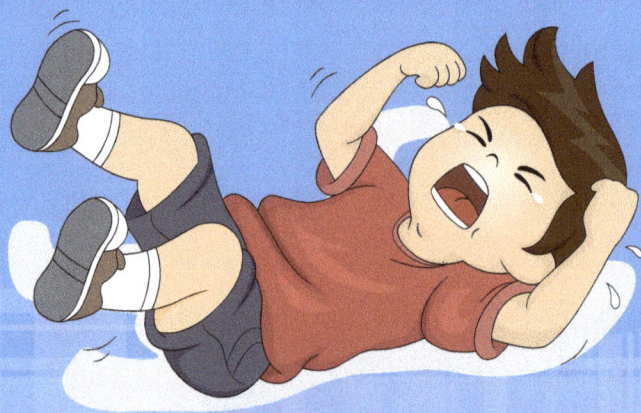

Teachers have many responsibilities. They must develop a

positive social-emotional climate in the classroom. They build trusting, respectful relationships with each child. Teachers provide a supportive physical environment and a nurturing learning environment to meet the needs of the little ones. With these cornerstones in place as a classroom foundation, you can address each child's individual needs.

Why do children misbehave? Typically, there are two main functions of behavior. The first is to get something such as an object, adult attention, or power. The other function of unwanted behavior is to get out of, or to avoid something such as a task or activity, a certain person or situation. For a child who is seeking attention by misbehaving, negative attention is better than no attention at all.

There is always a reason for misbehavior. Finding out the "why" of the behavior helps you to then figure out ways to address the situation. When a child is non-compliant on a regular basis, employ the ABC's of recording behavior described earlier.

The most important thing to remember is that all behavior is communication. Sometimes young children are telling you things through behavior that they don't have the skills, or language to communicate otherwise. Some of the messages you might be getting are "I'm bored," "I am overwhelmed," "You are asking too much of me," "I need you to teach me," or "I need your attention and support."

It is helpful as we look at non-compliance issues to record information about the antecedent, specific behavior and then the consequence. Seeing information in black and white can help give you a more objective picture of what is really going on, especially if you find the child's behavior very frustrating. For example, it may seem to you that Darius throws tantrums "all the time," but when you actually record the incidents, you may find it's really only three times a week. That's a very different reality.

Having objective information down on paper is helpful if you choose to include parents in your process (and, indeed, you should). It is beneficial for other professionals you may work with later in the child's program. As you examine your data, think very carefully about what the child may be getting out of the situation. What situation, place or person seems to be triggering the behavior? What does the behavior actually look like? What is the consequence? What happens right after the behavior? What steps can you take to allow the child to get what he needs in more appropriate ways, and to work within the boundaries of what is acceptable to you?

Having some information down in black and white will help you make more objective decisions about what the child is gaining from the behavior. Your written record will help you see what the child needs, and then start to take steps to offer more appropriate behaviors. The alternative behaviors should allow the child to get what he needs, working within the boundaries of what is acceptable to you.

Here are some examples of possible situations you might see in a classroom. Think about what the antecedent (what happens right before the behavior), the behavior itself and the consequences, (whether intentional or accidental) are.

Although Kinsley is quite verbal, she has a very hard time taking the perspective of others. If a child picks up a toy she loves, she will kick and punch them. She screams if she is not first in line every day.

Ralph is a child who is extremely sensitive to loud environments. Too much chaos, movement and noise is just overwhelming. When the music teacher leads the singing in her loud voice and plays her loud piano, the auditory stimulation is too much for Ralph. He has learned that when he misbehaves (not singing, pinching and poking others, creating a scene in general) the aide will take him out of the room. Even though he gets in trouble for his behavior, it's worth it to Ralph as he gets to escape that situation.

Trevor finds the 45-minute circle time that Miss Take conducts in her classroom far too long. (Check your developmentally appropriate expectations, Miss Take). Trevor has decided to remedy that situation by misbehaving each circle time so he can create some distraction and excitement for himself as well as for the rest of the class, because Miss Take is not.

Erin is a child with many language delays. She has trouble with receptive language, which means that she has a hard time processing all the words the teacher says as she reads a story to the group. She gets easily bored during the story because the words become meaningless to her, and then she refuses to stay in her seat.

Clayton has a hard time in line with his four-year-old classmates. He struggles with body awareness, so does not always know that he is too close to others and is too hands-on with them. He gets in trouble for this, but doesn't even realize what he is doing until it's too late. His friends don't want to stand by him in line.

Shawn's parents are headed for a bitter divorce. He has been watching a lot of angry arguments at home, has seen a couple of things thrown, and knows there is tension in the air. He is completely overwhelmed by the sudden lack of safety and security with his parents, and has become angry and defiant at school with teachers, especially when they become very directive with him. He doesn't realize it, but he is hoping to gain some power over his chaotic life. When he gets defiant, the teacher uses her angry voice which escalates him further.

Nathan has a diagnosis of autism. He has a hard time picking up on social cues, and needs very clear, simple directions. When the teacher is unclear in her directions, saying things like "take a seat," Nathan is confused and sometimes has trouble following directions, which frustrates his teacher. When Nathan gets very confused, he just shuts down completely.

There is no one-size-fix-all for defiant preschoolers and young children. However, by being a good observer of the situation, you can begin to assess what might be really going on, and what each child is trying to communicate through this behavior.

🔑 KEY POINTS

- All behaviors are driven by a need.
- Misbehaviors may be aimed at seeking something or avoiding something.
- The ABC method of recording behavior may help you to examine the causes of specific behaviors.
- All behavior is an attempt to communicate something.

Large, well-controlled studies show us that teachers can have a significant effect on children's behavior through the use of reinforcement techniques. **Reinforcement Theory of Motivation,** developed by B. F. Skinner, is highly regarded in the field of education. [10] For this system to work for you, you need to have a basic understanding of the theory.

As described by Skinner, **reinforcers** are basically rewards for a behavior. This can be any type of behavior, from social greetings to task completion. [10] Some reinforcers are positive and some are negative. It is important to understand that a negative reinforcer is not the same thing as a punishment. A good program will be built on a mixture of positive and negative reinforcement, but will not include punishments.

A **positive reinforcer** is something *given to* a learner to increase a certain behavior. A **negative reinforcer** is *something taken* away which in turn increases the desired behavior. For example, allowing a child to play with a favored toy when he completes a certain task is a positive reinforcement and will likely result in him completing the task again the next time it is presented.

On the other hand, removing a stimulus when a task is completed is negative reinforcement and should be seen as a reward also. If a child hates the feel of sticky dirty hands and you take him to go wash his hands, that is a negative reinforcer. You are *removing* something (the dirt from his hands) which is perceived by him as being a reward for washing. Negative reinforcement is not punishment. It is simply rewarding the child by removing something negative from the environment.

The reinforcer you choose for a child must be something that is rewarding to that child. One child may love stickers and will work hard to be awarded his sticker for the day. Another little one may care nothing about stickers, so that would not motivate him. Caleb's favorite reinforcer was fishing worms; Lane was rewarded by being allowed to wear an astronaut Halloween costume for a period of time. The reinforcer *has* to be motivating for the child, and it may change over time. A reinforcer may be time spent with a favored toy, a favorite person, or a favorite activity. When the child works for five minutes, perhaps he wins one minute to play with the little truck he likes. He only gets the favorite truck after working. You will need to figure out what is reinforcing for each child. Most typical children are motivated by social praise. They are happy to have a word or a look from the teacher that shows they have pleased you. It is rewarding for them to know that you approve of the work they just completed or the behavior they are exhibiting.

However, children with autism are not usually motivated by social praise. They may not respond to praise at all in the beginning. A child with autism often lacks the desire to please others. He will accomplish a task as a means to an end, but not just to please you. He may complete the job because he is interested in it, because he desires the end reward, because he wants to avoid the consequence of not completing the chore, or because he knows that it will help bring the session to an end if he complies with your request. Continue to praise and encourage him, even as you reward him with the object of choice. By pairing the social praise with the tangible reward, he should eventually get to the point that he understands the social praise. At this point the praise can become a reinforcer for the work he has done. This may take time, but it will be an important progression.

Undesired behavior may ultimately take the form of a **tantrum** or a meltdown. Lately many parents have adopted the term **"meltdown"** when their children are throwing good old fashioned temper tantrums. They seem to feel it is more socially acceptable to describe it as a meltdown. They may feel that their parental skills are less at risk of being judged when the child has a meltdown compared to throwing a temper tantrum. As a teacher, you need to learn to tell the difference between the two situations and handle them differently. Tantrums are triggered by something that the child wants, or wants to avoid. It is driven by the goal that he has in mind. He will keep checking your reaction to the behavior to see if he is making his point. If his audience stops paying attention to him, the tantrum subsides because there is no point to it. The tantrum resolves when he has attained his goal. Unfortunately, attaining the goal by throwing a tantrum increases the chances of the same behavior occurring the next time the child wants something.

Meltdowns are a totally different behavior even though they may look like tantrums to an uninformed observer. A meltdown occurs when a child is over-stressed or overwhelmed due to sensory or communication issues. A meltdown will continue whether or not the child has an audience. There is little you can do to intervene which will help him resolve the meltdown. Fatigue will set in, and you must be aware that safety becomes an issue because he may have no judgment during this fury. In contrast to a tantrum, the meltdown is not goal driven. He is not doing this because he wants something or wants to avoid something. This is happening because he is totally overwhelmed or over-stressed. While it is not driven by wants, you may indeed need to assist him to regain control. While tantrums are normally of fairly short duration, meltdowns can last for hours. This behavior is not dependent on having an audience, while a tantrum does depend on an audience. As one parent put it, "A typical child may throw a tantrum for five minutes because he wants a piece of candy, whereas my ASD child will have a meltdown for four hours because he heard the sound of water running."

In summary, behaviors fill a need for the child. Do not fear the meltdowns. They will happen. Just be armed with a plan of how you will handle the situation, while continuing to educate a classroom full of other children. Structure the environment to avoid the meltdowns if possible, but when they happen, calmly handle it and move on. (See the Sharing Our Strategies section of this book). Many of the behaviors of a child with autism are caused by too little or too much stimuli in one or more of the senses. Once you can figure out the driving cause, it will reduce your caregiver burden as you provide an alternate behavior to meet the need.

KEY POINTS

- A positive reinforcer is something given to the child to increase the chance that the behavior will happen again.
- A negative reinforcer is something that is removed from the child that increases the chance that he will want to repeat the behavior.
- Children with autism are often not motivated by social praise, so you must determine what does motivate him.
- A meltdown is different from a temper tantrum.

Chapter 5
Understanding and Accommodating

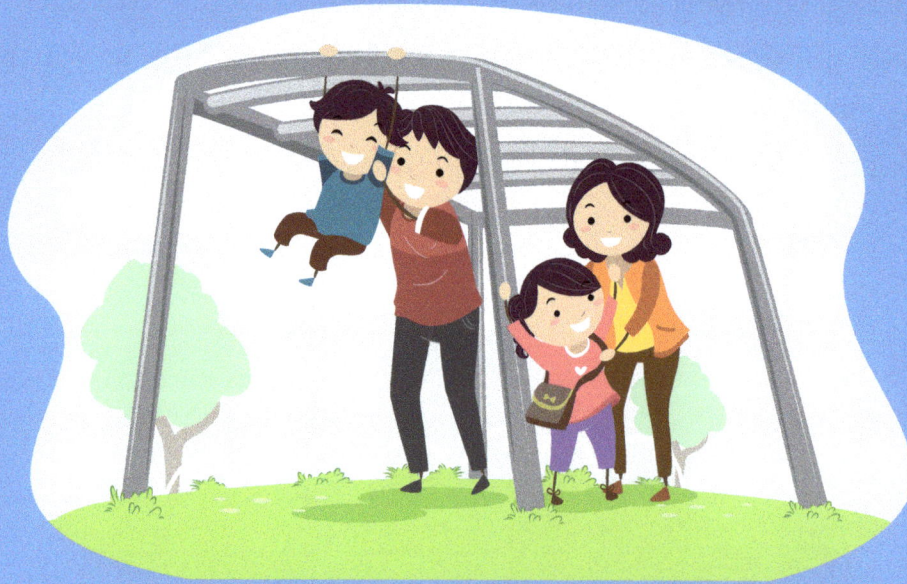

"Fair doesn't mean giving everybody the same thing. Fair means giving everybody what they need to succeed" (Rick Lavoie, 2001).

There is a delicate balance between accommodating and "giving in."

When we talk about making accommodations for children, the concern always comes up questioning how much is too much. "If I do all that, aren't I just giving in to him?" That's a valid question. When you think about accommodation in terms of the picture above, it makes more sense.

As teachers, we easily fall into the "fair" trap. Our own kids at home, as well as our kids at school have learned that crying, "It's not fair!" can be the magic words that play on adult guilt and get them what they want. In actuality, it's a little more complicated than that. Sometimes we do have to stack the deck a little or change things up somewhat to help a child succeed. It may be setting a different expectation, it may be providing more **scaffolding** help, it may be allowing something really important to the child to be a part of their day, but as long as we are helping children succeed, that's the definition of *fair*. If you explain to your typically developing students why Brandon always needs a certain cushy seat at circle time, or why Braxton gets to hold a tiny stuffed dog on the way outside, you will be amazed at the level of understanding shown by children. It's all in how you explain things, and in doing so kindly and honestly, you are not only helping your special needs child, you are helping others to learn.

Jan Luck and Dr. Barboa have written a series of books to help children understand autism. *Albert is My Friend: Helping Children Understand Autism* is a delightful read-aloud book for children in the early childhood age group. [11] It is available in four languages. You can follow that up by reading several other books in the series. Each book has a curriculum guide available to give you other activities to reinforce the lessons of diversity. Through the program of Early Acceptance Education©, understanding and acceptance of all is taught. If children learn early to accept the differences in one another, bullying and teasing can be significantly diminished. The more you work to build a sense of community and belonging in your classroom, the less teasing and unkindness you will see. People (even adults) don't tend to pick on those whom they see as a part of their own community. The more you build a classroom where all members are welcomed, valued and respected, the more positive relationships you will see among peers. You will watch your classroom society work to protect its more vulnerable members. Another great classroom resource is the book, *We Are All Stars*, by Mary Lou Datema, which promotes the acceptance of individual differences in the early childhood classroom. [12] When you reinforce the idea that different can be okay, you are giving all the children in your classroom a valuable life lesson.

Don't be afraid to try to some different **accommodations** to see if they help. If you don't try, you'll never know, and sometimes simple changes make a big difference. A cushion in the seat of a chair, a child's camping chair instead of a traditional classroom chair, or even a laundry basket to sit in are all perfectly acceptable examples of seating accommodations. Some children love the feel of a tube sock filled with rice or beans to give it weight and may want this across their shoulders or in their laps. Keep in mind that you may need to try something several times to see if it's effective.

Not every child in your classroom has to complete every activity every time. If a child does well for the first 5 minutes of circle time, and then is *done*, increase the time slowly to enable him to be a part of the entire experience. Allow the child to leave after 5 minutes and then build up slowing to staying longer. Holding a particular toy as the child makes transitions from one room to another is perfectly fine, as long as it helps. Holding a quiet "stimmy" or small object during a long assembly or while a special visitor is in the class is fine. If a child needs to leave the room for a few minutes to take a walk, go get a drink, or "help you" by delivering a message to another teacher, that's acceptable. Always observe the rules of the school and safety precautions in regard to child supervision.

Some children benefit by pushing a heavy box, or heavily loaded toy shopping cart down a hallway. Occupational therapists call this "heavy work," and that's okay if it helps the child calm himself and focus. If a child handles playing in shaving cream better by pushing a toy car through it rather than immersing her hands, or if she can't handle the texture of wet spaghetti, but will play in other wet sensory materials, that's okay.

Just like other adults in the community sometimes tiptoe around what to say or not to say around a child with a disability, teachers struggle with how much or what to say in the classroom. If you want to build a classroom community, you can't shy away from questions, and you need to be able to explain why you are making accommodations for some in your classroom. Brody was completely overwhelmed by sitting in the middle of the group at circle time; that was just too much togetherness for him. However, he did fine sitting at the end of the circle time rainbow of chairs. The teacher explained to the class that being in the middle was hard for Brody and that they could help Brody by always allowing him to sit in the chair at the end. The next day as the group gathered for circle time, one student called Brody to his chair while another guarded it and made sure nobody else sat there.

The importance of explaining and guiding your students to understanding is, of course, not just relevant to their classmates with autism. Brooks had some serious scarring on his legs from an accident when he was very young; he was completely unaffected by the look of his legs and often wore shorts. The second day he was in class, another student asked him what had happened to his legs. When Brooks told him, the other child responded with "Oh," and that was the end of that. It didn't come up again. You will find that if you tell your students why Amanda needs to sit on the squishy seat, (it helps her to be a better listener) why Cody likes to hold a toy dog at group time (it helps him not to feel nervous) or why Quintan sometimes has meltdowns, (he is working on learning self- control and how to solve problems) your other students will understand and support you and that child. Explanations can be simple and short. Remind your students that everybody is learning something; some are learning to write their names; some are learning letters or shapes; some are learning to follow directions; some are learning to use their words. Nobody knows everything and none of us ever will. We just help each other along the journey as well as we can!

🔑 KEY POINTS

- "Fair" means giving each child what he needs to succeed.
- Early Acceptance Education© can increase tolerance and reduce bullying.
- Don't shy away from explaining to the class what accommodations you are making for some and why. We are all learning, all the time.

There are legalities that teachers must be aware of which assure a child is provided with what he needs. If a child has been tested, has been diagnosed with a disability and has been given an individual learning plan with specific goals and accommodations to help with learning, that child now has an **Individual Education Plan (IEP)**. If he is less than three years old, the agency evaluating him will have generated an **Individualized Family Service Plan (IFSP)** if services are warranted.

If you are a public school teacher, be aware that an IEP is a legal document. The accommodations you must provide your student are dictated to you by the IEP. Professionals, parents and others who serve the child coordinate to come up with the best individualized plan for the child based on test results and current functioning. IEP meetings can be strenuous, but the best child-centered IEP is arrived at when all sides work together. The strategies and modifications listed on this document are non-negotiable. Neither are they choices. It is important for you to know that by law, you must follow the directives listed on the document if you are working in a public school. In addition to special education minutes the child receives, the IEP may lay out classroom modifications, curricular modifications and how you may or may not discipline this child. It lists a current level of functioning and will identify exactly what this child needs to develop academically and socially.

If you are working in a child care setting, the parents should be able to provide you a copy of the IEP. A private child care setting is not mandated to follow the dictates of the IEP in the same way the public school system is, but doing so is considered "best practice' and will surely help your student succeed. With parental permission, you should be able to contact public school members of the team, and often private therapists as well to gain additional knowledge and insight into how best to serve this child. Take advantage of the opportunity to speak with these highly trained people who can give you lots of information about that child and about autism in general. Private schools have no legal obligation to follow the IEP or the IFSP.

The idea in working with any child on the autism spectrum is to scaffold behaviors and skills toward "typical" as much as possible. For some children, this won't be very hard; for some it will be an ongoing, lifelong challenge. Take comfort in the fact that if you have a child with a diagnosis of autism or who is on a current IEP, you have a team to help you answer specific questions and help you with learning strategies tailored toward that child. Be sure to talk with the most important members of the team, the child's parents, about expectations and strategies at home. Understand that some sensory, communication or cognitive needs may always be present. The key is to focus on those life skills that will be most important for the child. This is where the balance comes in. Have high expectations for the child and anticipate that he will participate in regular activities as much as possible.

Dallas hated math in first grade and had worked hard to throw tantrums at math time to escape having to stay in class. His astute teacher recognized what was going on and had a Prepchat© with him about math class, including what he would learn and what her expectations were. She explained to the class that Dallas was learning to be a worker, and that if he got upset, they were not to worry, she would help Dallas with his learning. She allowed Dallas a stimmy to hold in his pocket (more about Prepchats© and stimmies later) but also told him that he would be expected to do his share of the work in class. The teacher felt that Dallas was using his behaviors to manipulate an escape from work. He was not leaving due to overstimulation, but as a way to get away from the math. She told Dallas he would not be allowed to leave the room again during math. Her very clear communication on the subject worked, and, although Dallas still didn't enjoy math, he understood the teacher was not willing to give in on this one. That's the tricky part, and where your team can help you in determining what your realistic expectations should be.

We are all working constantly, often without realizing it, to reach a state of equilibrium- or a comfort zone, with our bodies. We each need just enough sensory input, but not too much. When you tap your pencil on the table during a class, avoid getting your fingers in sticky syrup, chew gum to keep yourself awake in church, remove yourself from loud music at a party, or avoid looking at a person standing in front of a sunlit window, you are working to provide yourself with just the right amount of visual, aural (sound), oral and tactile input. Think of it this way; everybody has a "cup" just for sensory input. If you have a very small "cup", it may not take much input for you to fill your "cup" and then not want more. If you have a large "cup", it may take a lot of sensory input to reach the state of equilibrium, and you may spend a lot of time looking for things that can help you fill your "cup".

Observing your children will help you to notice any sensory needs they are displaying. Utilizing your ABC recording chart to observe and document behaviors more closely will enhance the classroom management. [6] A great teacher is one who recognizes the individual sensory needs of students and tries to accommodate those needs. Knowing that children with autism often have some sensory needs will help you with planning for learning activities and anticipating potential difficulties. It's part of understanding our students. It's no biggie!

KEY POINTS

- IEPs and IFSPs are legal documents that must be followed.
- Scaffold the teaching of social skills and behaviors to reach goals.
- A good teacher plans for individual learning differences.

Communication Strategies

Every day you work with children you will be teaching communication skills in multiple ways. These skills are among the most important skills you will be giving to the children in your care. While we normally think of spoken language as the main goal in teaching communication, there are many functional forms of getting a message from one person to another. When you are working with children with special needs, spoken language may not be your first goal. You may need to look at other, alternative methods of developing language. Do not worry that by using other means of communication you will delay the onset of spoken language. Research shows that quite the opposite is true. Using some basic sign language or speaking devices actually helps develop spoken language. If you and your professional team can give the child a means to communicate basic wants and needs, you are relieving him of the frustrations that result from not being understood. By providing him with this skill you will be avoiding behavior issues.

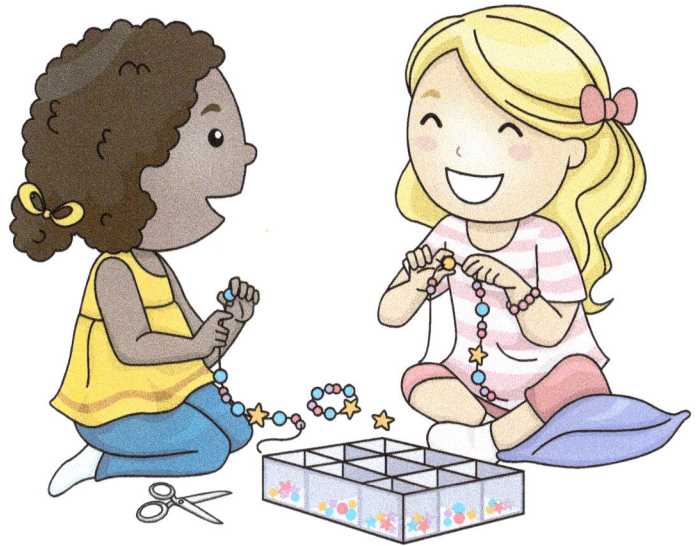

Some preschoolers who have autism may not even be capable of communicating in any fashion at a high enough level to have their needs met. One of the first things you must begin to give the child is a way to express himself. No academic teaching can begin until you reduce the frustration.

Working with the parents and the speech-language pathologist, your team will determine the best way to begin to teach the child to communicate. If you decide to begin with a nonverbal approach, you will have the choice of low tech or high tech methods. Low tech options range from the use of simple cue cards to a Picture Exchange Communication System (PECS®), which requires full teacher training. [13] If you opt for a high tech system, choices range from a simple app on the iPad to expensive, complex commercially available devices. In making the decision of which type of communication to teach the child, you will need to consider his age and his skill level. While even preschoolers can manage the use of basic technology, the decision of whether or not to employ that method is a complicated one, and will involve input from all of the professionals working with the child, as well as the parents.

Sign language can be a quick easy way to give the child a means of communicating. This does not necessarily mean that you will need to rush out and learn a formal system of sign language. You may begin with a few broad gestures, and later refine and expand the list. Many people prefer to start with the use of basic signs because of the simple benefits to a child with autism. You can start using signs without buying any expensive equipment. Use of basic signs has been shown to improve eye contact in children with autism, because they must look to you to see the sign you are teaching them. Signing has the added benefit of decreasing echolalia, which is verbalization that may interfere with the true communication in children with autism. Another benefit of using signs as compared to an electronic device is that they can be used in the home, classroom, or on the playground. Whereas a device may need to be protected from rough play, and is useless if not charged, sign language is consistent and reliable.

Most people begin with a couple of easy, general signs, such as "more" or "please." For other children with autism, those signs are too abstract and should be replaced by more concrete signs, such as "water." Whichever signs you choose, move forward and continue to add signs as the child masters them. Signs that will be particularly helpful include signs for the names of his family members and the sign for "toilet." A good method for teaching the basic signs is the hand-over-hand method. Simply hold his hands and form the sign while you verbalize the words. Be patient as you make these connections for him. If you begin with some easy basic signs, as time passes, in most cases you will likely use those skills as a bridge to oral communication.

One huge benefit of using early sign language is that it is free, compared to the very expensive high tech devices. Sign language promotes social skills better than the use of a communication device does. You may find that signing encourages eye contact more than an electronic device can. It has the benefit of decreasing echolalia, or repetitive language, and helps develop a relationship between the child and the caregiver. Just be sure to coordinate the signs you decide to use between all the people who care for the child, so home and school are working together.

There are multiple systems of sign language. If you are working with a speech-language pathologist, consult with her to determine the system of most benefit to the child. To determine which method you will use, the SLP could help you consider the child's age level and skill level to choose the most appropriate system. The SLP can train you in the use of the technique chosen. Always check with the family to see if any systems are already in place through other therapies, and see how the family communicates at home.

High tech systems, on the other hand, can sometimes be programmed with a human voice that can be understood by anyone in the child's environment, even strangers. Children often have a strong interest in electronic gadgets and that may be a motivation. Little ones can actually learn to use the devices faster than they learn sign language, but those who use the devices are slower to transition to oral speech than those who begin with signs.

The high tech devices do have certain advantages. Many early learners will benefit from a communication device, but those have drawbacks to consider. They need to be charged or they are useless. Using a device requires carrying it from place to place as they navigate their environments. High tech devices may be impossible to use on the playground. Because of the positive and negative aspects of each method of communication, you might decide to use a combination of methods. For example, you could use a communication device in the classroom, and sign language when he is on the playground.

If your choice is to use an electronic device, please do not allow gaming on the same device that the child uses for communication. These two functions must be kept separate, on two distinctively different devices, or the child will be continually wanting to play games on his communication device. After endless begging by her child to play a game on his communication device, Kristen gave in and allowed it "just once". She forever regretted that moment.

No matter what method you choose to use when communicating with a child on the autism spectrum, some consistencies will apply. For example, whether you use signs, devices or oral language, avoid using all- inclusive words, such as *"always, never, no one, everyone, all or none."* Sentences that contain these words will be confusing to children on the spectrum, because they will take it very literally, and will think of scenarios to prove you wrong. Once they figure out a scenario to disprove the rule, you will lose credibility.

The strategies used to develop functional language will have similarities as you teach the child. One basic strategy for improving the child's language is **expansion.** This consists of repeating an immature sentence formed by a child, expanding the idea in the process. For example, if a child sees a dog and exclaims "See doggie!" you can encourage his language development by answering, "We see a big brown dog!" Another example would be if the child says "Mommy go," you could answer with "Mommy goes to work and you go to school."

Another technique that is recommended to improve a child's language is known as **revision.** In this strategy, the teacher repeats the immature sentence spoken by the child, discretely stressing the corrected version. For example, if the child says, "I drinked the milk," say "Yes, you *drank* the milk." If the child says, "I falled down," repeat, "You *fell* down."

Young children on the autism spectrum will need to be actually taught language skills that typical children just pick up naturally by watching others. This includes pointing, asking for help, complimenting others, social greetings and conversation starters. Thanking others is a social skill picked up at a young age by most children. However, for the ASD child, this is a difficult concept. If you tell him to "Say thank you," he will likely ask why. He may even be blunt and ask why he has to say thank you for something he does not like, or thinks is ugly. To teach children these communication skills, you will need to prompt him to greet others, to give a compliment, to thank others, and to ask for help. Teach him how to respond when others give him a compliment. **Role playing** is a helpful technique for teaching these skills.

Conversation skills in general will need to be taught. Children must learn to take turns in a conversation. This is difficult to learn, but so important as they go through life. Many people with autism continue to plow through their own one-sided conversation while the others around them interact with one another in a social conversation. Many of them do not know when to stop talking or how to follow a topic as it shifts from one line of conversation to another. They simply must be taught. Help them follow the conversation by asking questions to keep them on track with the others.

When teaching young children, keep in mind that the skill of following directions is learned in steps. First, the child must understand how to follow a single directive. Only when that is mastered can he understand how to follow a two part, then a three-part command. If you present a three-part directive to a child who is just learning to follow a simple command, you are setting him up for failure and frustration. Break it down. For example, rather than saying, "Hang up your coat, get your book and sit down," simplify it. Say, "Hang up your coat." When that has been accomplished, add, "Get your book." When he has done this, tell him, "Sit down." As the child begins to show success following a single direction, begin giving him a two step command using two related directives. For example, "Take off your coat and hat." After he masters a two step command referring to two related items, begin to introduce two step commands containing two unrelated items, such as, "Take off your coat, then get a drink."

Directives given to children are more successful if you give them in the form of a statement rather than a question. Instead of saying "Do you want to pick up those toys now?" say, "Pick up the toys." Rather than saying, "Are you ready for circle time?" say, "Come to the carpet for circle time." Don't fall into the habit of asking the child, "Okay?" at the end of each sentence, unless you really do intend to give him a choice. An example of this is the teacher who says, "We are going to put our coats on now, okay?" Simply tell him. Don't ask him if it is "okay" with him unless you really want to know his opinion of your request.

Another helpful strategy is to state directions in the positive rather than the negative. Tell them what you *want* them to do rather than what you *don't want* them to do. For example, say, "Walk," instead of saying, "Don't run!" Children often have short attention spans and short memories. They may only remember the last word they heard, which was "run." If you tell them, "Don't run," they may think they are pleasing you when they take off running. When you tell an early learner what NOT to do, he may have no idea of what behavior you actually WANT from them. Reducing the negative wording increases a happy environment for the class.

Directives must be very clear. If your student is not responding to you as you give a directive, try rephrasing it using more exact language. Rather than saying, "It's time to go now," try saying, "It is time for us to get on the bus to go home." Whether giving a directive or asking a question, allow extra time for children with ASD to process what he hears. This student may take longer than a typical child to respond. Give him time to respond or to answer before piling on more demands.

Excessive questioning is common in children on the spectrum. They may even ask the same question continuously. Your challenge is to determine why the behavior is occurring. Is he really seeking the answer and forgetting it that quickly, or does he just want your attention and this is the only way he knows to get it?

By careful observation of the child, you will discover things that are motivating to him. Pay attention to what motivates and reinforces his actions. Watch which toys he prefers and use those in your communication plans. If you place his favorite toys on the top shelf where he can see them but cannot reach them, this will motivate him to communicate his desires to you. Children are resourceful and may even catch onto this and attempt to sabotage your good intentions. Kennedy was a nonverbal girl who loved playing with a specific toy truck. When the class went out to recess, one teacher routinely stayed behind to tidy the room. Kennedy soon caught on that she would be required to ask for her favorite truck when she returned from recess, so she started hiding it in an accessible place as recess time approached.

If a child lacks a functional form of communication, his behaviors become his means of communication. If the teachers and parents don't understand what the child is trying to tell them, there is a high potential that the child will become frustrated and act out, or simply withdraw and give up in his attempts to communicate.

🔑 KEY POINTS

- Revision is a strategy in which the teacher repeats the immature sentence spoken by the child, discretely stressing the corrected version.
- Expansion is a strategy that consists of repeating an immature sentence formed by a child, expanding the idea in the process.
- State directions as a sentence, not as a question.
- State directions in the positive rather than the negative.
- There are many ways to communicate. Oral speech is just one method.
- High tech and low tech devices both have their pros and cons.
- The use of simple sign language promotes the development of oral speech.

Strategies for Teaching Social Skills

One of the most important tasks of childhood is to learn how to get along with other people. This is the time of life when little ones figure out how to interact with others. They must learn how to get along with different classifications of people. The expectation of how to act with another four-year-old child is different from the way that they should act toward an adult. The social interactions they are learning will enable them to make friends throughout life. It is essential for them to learn how to establish friendships. As we go through life, it is important to have friends. Friends become our support group, and a source of happiness for us. They help us cope with stressful situations, and they share our happiness when good things happen. Children with special needs will need extra guidance in learning how to develop and maintain friendships.

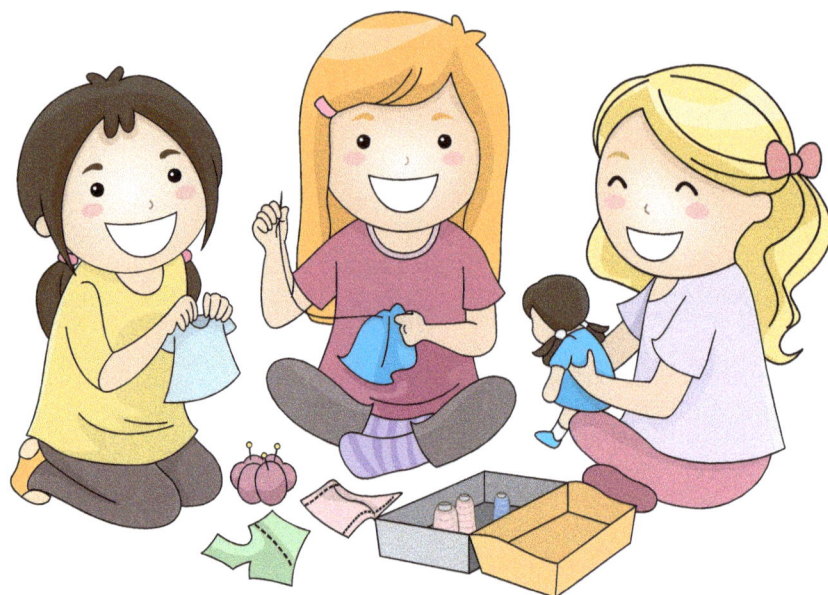

A prominent feature of autism is difficulty with social situations. The things that typical people do to regulate those social interactions may be deficit in people with ASD. Nonverbal behaviors such as eye contact and facial expressions play a role in regulating social behaviors. Because they have difficulty interpreting these signs, they may fail to develop peer relationships at an appropriate level. You may notice a lack of spontaneity in sharing social enjoyment. You may note poor social reciprocity. A typical child will pick up these skills by observing the adults in his environment. Children on the spectrum will need to actually be taught how to get along with others and form friendships. You will teach them how to read facial and body language. You will teach them how to make and keep friends. Showing an interest in others must be fostered and they must learn to nurture relationships.

The difficulty that a child with ASD displays in social situations must be addressed from both sides of the problem. Not only will you need to help this child learn social conventions, you will also need to teach the other children in the classroom how to play with that particular child. By explaining why he reacts to situations in a particular manner, you can help the children understand the unusual behaviors. By teaching the class at a young age that differences between people are okay, you can actually have a profound effect on their lives. Learning acceptance of diverse people in the preschool years can prevent bullying in later years. This is an ongoing process for typically developing children as well. They must learn all the social subtleties of working with someone who is very different from themselves. Typical children may say or do inappropriate things in the process of learning social skills. Most likely, they are not trying to be mean or unkind; they are learning how to get along in society. That's a different situation than a child who intentionally bullies.

Problems with social skills that you may observe include a lack of being able to see things from another person's point of view, poor conversational skills, poor eye contact, lack of understanding, and a poor sense of humor. These children often model their behaviors after adults in their environment rather than imitating their peers.

Because they have trouble learning social skills, this population is often naive or immature compared to their classmates. They may innocently reach up and touch the teacher's breasts as they are talking to her, not understanding that such behavior is socially inappropriate. They may actually need to be taught that this behavior is inappropriate, whereas a typical child already has that understanding by this age.

The social skill of understanding when someone is kidding them will need to be taught.

They are so literal in their understanding that when someone teases, kids, or makes a joke, they will think it is the truth. When this occurs you will need to guide them toward understanding. An example of this is when Kate picks up a toy wand and puts on a little tiara and proclaims, "I am a princess." As the other children run to join in the fun, Braden gets angry and insists, "Kate said she is a princess and she is *lying*! She is just a girl!"

Another social factor you will notice is that children with autism are usually very honest. While this is commendable in most situations, it can interfere with social interactions in other situations. As the children all complete an art project, this child is likely to give a very truthful and frank opinion about the product made by others. You may hear him judge another child's paintings with the words, "That is ugly." He may even give his unsolicited opinion that the other child is ugly or fat. The child on the spectrum views this as being honest, and has no filter to remind him to be kind or socially appropriate in sharing his opinions.

The honesty factor is further complicated by the fact that the truth they share is the truth from their own immature perspective. As George Costanza proclaims on the *Seinfeld* sitcom, "It's not a lie if you believe it." [14]

It may be helpful to have puppets in your classroom to help demonstrate appropriate social skills. You can take an individual picture of every child in your classroom, make these into puppets (either tape the pictures to popsicle sticks or stand them in large binder clips) and use them to role play social situations. Enlist the help of peers in the classroom to help teach and role play specific situations. Having a puppet of every classmate is a great community building opportunity as well. You will find all of your little ones enjoying the puppets. Be sure to make a puppet of each adult the children work with as well.

One reason social skills are lacking is that the child with autism has often had less opportunity to practice getting along with others, as he may be more isolated in his home life. Many parents of special needs children avoid taking them to social functions or gatherings, due to experiences they have encountered. They may have had bad experiences with judgmental looks or unkind words from other parents at the park playground, at church, or at birthday parties. It becomes easier and less painful to plan family activities that do not include outings, resulting in less social exposure for the child. With patience and understanding for the trauma a child may be feeling, the teacher can help him become more a part of the social world.

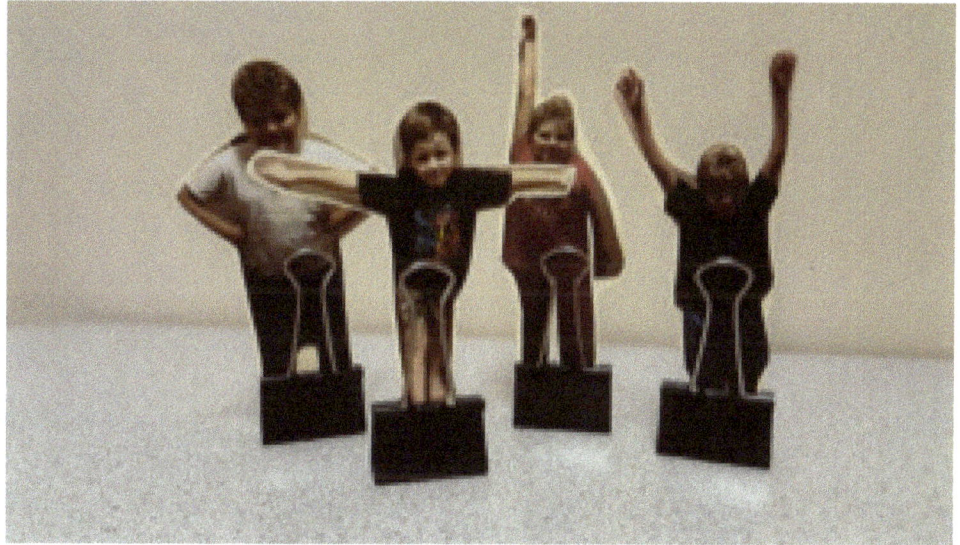

🔑 KEY POINTS

- Teaching children to get along with one another is one of your most important tasks.
- Children with autism often have difficulty in social skills. While some children on the spectrum prefer to play alone, others crave social intereaction, but lack the needed skills.
- The other children in the class must be taught how to get along with the special needs children.
- Children with ASD often do not understand teasing or kidding.

PART THREE
TEACHING TECHNIQUES

Chapter 6
Learning Activities

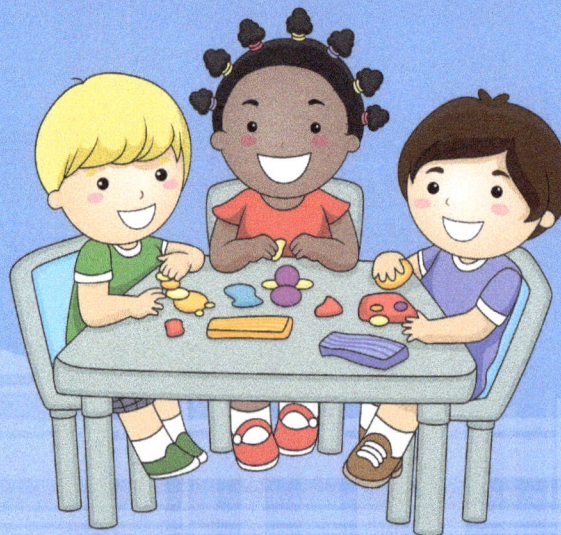

Play

There are many approaches to teaching. Small children respond better to some strategies than they do to others. Teaching through play is the most fun, yet highly effective way to teach young children.

Children progress through a hierarchy of types of play. Lower functioning or pre-verbal children with autism spend much of their time engaged in solitary play. They may even be noted to adjust their body position to exclude others from joining them. They seem to be protecting their personal space. When given a toy, they often do not play with it in the expected way. Instead, they may stare at it, especially at any moving parts. A typical child who picks up a toy car will run it on an imaginary road on the loor, the table, or even on the wall. The child with autism, however, may just enjoy looking at the toy from different angles, or watching the wheels spin. The object in his hand does not necessarily represent a car for him, but rather is an object of enchantment to be looked at intently.

The push in past years has been to encourage children toward functional play—that is, using objects such as toy cars in the way they are intended to be used. However, as we learn more about autism, we also recognize the need to be more accepting of all forms of play, including some of those activities that merely look repetitive and non-functional to us. After all, play should be something that brings enjoyment, and these activities are often enjoyable to our children on the spectrum. Each family and teacher will need to have a conversation about what play can and should look like for each child, and the extent to which the play can be scaffolded to become more interactive.

Preferring to play alone is a common trait of those with ASD. Sometimes they just don't enjoy being around others or need those connections. At other times, these children would like to play with others but just don't know how. We do know that if a child can learn to imitate others, the door is open to expedited learning. This is where the teacher's intervention can be more successful.

During play, the most basic lessons can be learned. He can learn to take turns, which facilitates joint attention. Joint attention is the communication between two people as they interact. He can learn to follow simple directions. He can learn basic concepts. Just exploring his environment while playing teaches him about his world. Playground experiences teach him about how his body moves in space and the relationship his body has to the earth. Those basic concepts are often more difficult for children with special needs. You may notice they are at a more fundamental level in their play activity, and they take longer to move through the stages. They might be playing at a noticeably lower level than their classmates. It is important to a child's cognitive level for him to progress through the stages of play. Children who do not have play skills are at a distinct disadvantage in the development of language and cognitive skills. Be patient and time will be your ally to help them progress to a higher, more productive level of play.

For those children who are lacking in play skills and don't know what to do with toys and materials, sometimes specific visuals can help. You may need to show them exactly what they can do with Play-Doh®, a Mr. Potato Head™ toy or blocks. While most children pick up ideas from watching and playing with others, children on the spectrum may not.

This visual gives a child very specific ideas of what can be done on a playground.

🔑 KEY POINTS

- Children can learn many basic lessons through play.
- Children on the spectrum often prefer to play alone.
- They may play with toys in unusual ways, often preferring to stare at moving parts of the toy.
- Children with ASD may need help to progress through the stages of play.

Here are some very specific building block ideas.

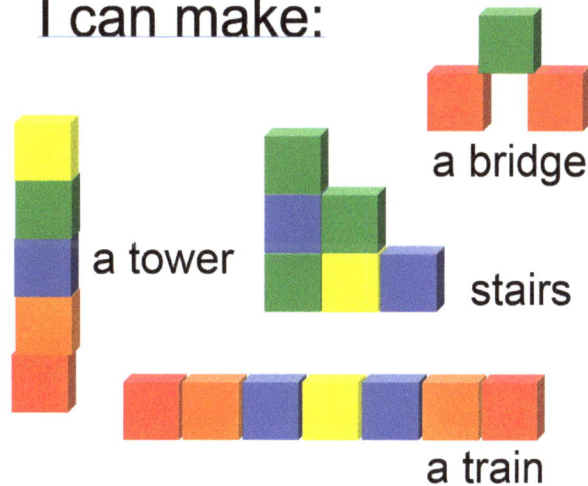

I can make:

a bridge

a tower

stairs

a train

Reading

Reading to the children is an important strategy, both with typical children and those with special needs. Read to them often. A child with special needs will not be able to sit and listen to a story as long as a typical child can. Maybe you can get his attention for a few seconds to show him an attractive picture along with a few words. Slowly work up. You have two real tasks here- to teach him to love books and reading, and to develop his pre-reading skills. Both of those will be important to his later academic success.

Children begin to acquire **pre-reading skills** long before they actually start to read. They learn that books have pages and we turn those pages as we read. They learn that pages contain pictures and words, and that we read the book from front to back, turning pages from right to left, one at a time. They learn about consistency of print, that the words remain the same every time the story is read. They learn that if you turn the book it will be upside down, and we cannot read it that way. All of the things they learn at this stage allow them to progress into early reading.

Choose books that have colorful, enchanting pictures. Don't offer a book that has too many words per page. It is imperative to choose books of high interest at this level. Ask easy questions as you go along, and have short discussions about the pictures in the book. Make reading a fun activity. Children love to hear you use animated, fun voices as you read. Young children enjoy books with photo. They enjoy reading the same book over and over because they like the predictability of knowing what comes next. Have fun when you read, and let them know that you are enjoying the book.

KEY POINTS

- Read to children often, choosing colorful, engaging books.
- Children learn pre-reading skills long before they actually start to read.
- Choose books of a high interest level and read in a lively, animated voice.

Prepchat© and the ChoicesChat©

There are books available to help teach important social skills, such *Hands Are Not For Hitting*[15] and *Words Are Not For Hurting*[16] (The Best Behavior Series, 2002-2004). When you teach an inclusive class, teaching social skills becomes very important. Even children who are basically pre-verbal will benefit from the social activities you introduce to the group. Two of the main strategies you can employ in teaching social skills are the **Prepchat**© and the **ChoicesChat**© described in the book *Tic Toc Autism Clock* (2015) by Barboa and Obrey.[5]

These two techniques apply to typical children as well as children with special needs.

PrepChats© and ChoicesChats© are totally individualized to each situation and require no expensive equipment. Prepare an individual child or the class as a whole to any social situation they are about to face. Keep your chat short and simple. The PrepChat© is your chance to provide them with a guideline of what to expect. You will include any rules for the upcoming situation and tell them what behavior you expect of them. As the class advances in understanding, you will modify the PrepChats© to meet their needs. When you have special needs children who may not be at the same cognitive level or social level as the rest of the class, you may give a short PrepChat© to the entire class and add a little PrepChat© directed more to the child who needs extra guidance. Here is an example of what this may look like:

We are going to walk to the lunch room.

We walk quietly in the hall.

We stay together in the hall.

When we get to the lunchroom we will sit at a table.

James, you will walk with Miss Pat.

You will keep your hands to yourself.

You will walk slowly.

The PrepChat© is short and calm and will help the child work through any upcoming situation that may cause him anxiety.

The ChoicesChat© is a little talk you have with the child after a situation has occurred. A ChoicesChat© is calm and instructional. If the child can respond to you, that is a good time to encourage his involvement. Use this teaching moment to examine the social error. Some children will need more coaching than others. At this time, you will involve a child in making a plan so that the social error does not happen again. A ChoicesChat© may look like this:

Teacher: Do you know why Aiden hit you?
Child: I took his car.

Teacher: Was it a good choice to take his car?
Child: No.

Teacher: What would be a better choice next time?
Child: I should not take Aiden's car.

Robert Havighurst, in his book *Human Development and Education* (1952), popularized the term "**teachable moments**"[17] While the term was originally meant to refer to the educational opportunities during traumatic or major episodes which occur in daily life, it can surely be applied to the continuing daily life when teaching young children. Every statement that you utter creates a teachable moment. Jan Luck, co-author of *Albert is My Friend; Helping Children Understand Autism* (2015), refers to this phenomenon as an "**ActionChat©**." [11]

The words you use, the tone of your voice, and the information given all teach children about the world around them. They are picking up your vocabulary and your grammar. They are learning how sentences are formed, as well as absorbing the information you are giving them. Understand the impact of every word you say and make the most of this teaching opportunity.

In two Head Start Centers the authors visited this week, we saw a perfect contrast between teachers who lost the teachable moment, and others who created beautiful ActionChats©. Both centers were practicing fire drills that day. In the first center, the unprepared children heard the alarm and looked around in confusion. The teacher calmly told the children to line up and go out the door. She led the children across the yard to the fence where she spent the next precious minutes doing a roll call. She encouraged each child to respond as she called their names, even though the three teachers standing there could clearly see who was present and would know if anyone was unaccounted for. They practiced saying, "Here" when their names were called, never being given a reason for this activity.

At the second center, Miss Marissa prepared the children with a well presented PrepChat©. She told them that they were going to hear a loud buzzing sound that we call a "fire drill." She explained step by step how they would line up and walk out the door. She told them the purpose of the fire drill. She reassured them of the fact that the teachers and director would keep them safe. When the fire drill sounded and the children arrived at the safety of the fence area, Miss Marissa was joined by the center director, Miss Renate. Miss Renate provided the children with a perfect ActionChat©. She told the children what was happening at the moment. She reinforced what Miss Marissa had told the youngsters in the PrepChat©. She taught them what would happen if there were really a fire, and who would come to help them. She reiterated the safety rules and what is expected of them when the fire drill rings. They were informed about how this exercise ends. She told them that after she checks the building to make sure it is all safe, she will tell Miss Marissa, and Miss Marissa will take the children back into the building. All of this took about the same amount of time as the fire drill in the class where they spent the whole time taking roll. Although the teachers in the first class were well meaning, they missed an important teachable moment.

Teachable moments are present all through the day for teachers who are eager to take advantage of an available moment. Miss Amy, a Head Start teacher, sits with her children through breakfast and lunch, as is the practice for that program. She is a brilliant teacher who knows that when their mouths are busy eating, she has access to their ears and thereby their brains. While the students eat, they are totally engaged listening to Miss Amy skillfully tell the story of the Gingerbread Boy or other favorite childhood tales. She is not standing in front of the class with a book, showing pictures and reading. She is spinning the tale as she remembers it, with vivid detail and enthusiasm and the children are riveted on her every word. As they eat, they listen quietly as Miss Amy paints mental pictures encouraging each child's imagination to grow.

Besides vocabulary and grammar, social skills are taught through modeling and prompting as children listen to you talk. Demonstrate for them that when we greet people we say, "Hi" or "Hello" or "Good morning." When we are leaving someone, show them through your own behavior that we say, "Goodbye." If this is not yet automatic for the child, prompt him to verbalize the greeting. If he cannot yet verbalize, prompt him to wave goodbye, even if it requires assisting him physically. A good way to promote language development is to combine the words with the motion such as waving bye-bye. Keep in mind that the special needs children in your class may well be operating on a lower level than the rest of the class, so you will need to individualize your prompts and modeling.

For most typical children, hearing a PrepChat© or an ActionChat© one time does not cement it in their minds. Most little ones need to hear the same information again and again in order to learn it. This is even more true of most children with autism. Information must be given to them many times before they truly have it stored in memory.

⚷ KEY POINTS

- Use PrepChats© to tell the child in a simple way what to expect.
- Use ActionChats© to make any moment a teachable moment.
- Use ChoicesChats© to discuss choices that a child has made.
- Children learn social skills by watching your actions.

Music and Movement

Teaching children should be fun for you and for the little ones. A good way to add fun into your day is the integration of music and movement activities. People who write commercials know that rhythm and melody are good ways to integrate something into our memories. We remember the commercial that includes a little jingle or a short song. Think about the way you learned your alphabet. You probably learned to sing the letters before you actually learned to say them. There are songs to teach the days of the week, counting skills, the colors and many other concepts. Some are associated with a little finger play. The song *Where is Thumbkin?* actually teaches children the social skill of greeting another (as well as sequencing, fine motor skills and language).

Another good way to increase learning is to add movement to the learning. In a book titled *Smart Moves: Learning is Not all in Your Head,* Dr. Carla Hannaford (1995), documents the relationship between movement and academic learning. [18] Children learn faster and have more fun learning if there is physical movement associated with the task. Movement is accepted as being beneficial to cognition.

When teaching children with autism, they must actually be taught how to learn. Be kind and gentle and teach through multiple rounds of repetition. It may literally take thousands of repetitions for a child to learn a single skill. Children with autism have more difficulty learning that the typical child does. It will require more patience from the teacher, but by understanding this fact, you are giving yourself the means to provide an effective education for the child.

🔑 KEY POINTS

- Adding music to a learning activity helps the child learn.
- Adding movement to a learning activity is a good technique.
- Children with autism must actually be taught how to learn.

Chapter 7

Your Teaching Bag of Tricks

Successful educators use teaching techniques that have been proven to be effective through large, well-controlled studies. Just as a bricklayer uses a trowel and cement to build a building, you will depend on your trusty tools to build your students' knowledge. A basic teaching toolbox contains strategies and techniques that you will learn to apply in your teaching every day. These tools are essential as you teach children with special needs. They will assure the consistency and excellence to enable you to perform at your best. As you incorporate each tool into your daily teaching, it will become second nature and will actually make your job easier. Among the important teaching tools you will use daily are:

1. Goal setting
2. Appropriate equipment
3. Predictability
4. Scheduling
5. Coping strategies for children
6. Task analysis
7. Rewards and reinforcers
8. Visual supports
9. Peer helpers
10. Pets

Goals

Setting goals is a good way to motivate both teacher and student. It is the tool you use to measure your outcomes, as you track your progress toward the goals you set. Goals are your roadmap to know where you are going each day. They keep your program on track and help you feel less fragmented. Modern corporations set goals for each of their employees, from managers on the top level to line level employees on the bottom ranks. Businesses generally base their goal structure on the fact that setting goals leads to increased performance.

Set goals that are neither too high, nor too low. They should be aggressive but achievable. Goals that are too high assure failure. Goals that are too low do not motivate the child. Set high goals, with small baby steps to reach those goals. Document your progress through small steps.

When you formulate your goals, do yourself and the child a favor. State the goal in *positive* rather than *negative* language. Rather than documenting what behavior will end, tell what behavior will emerge. For example, rather than saying that James will "stop hitting other children" state that he "will keep his hands to himself."

While you will usually have several goals for a child in any given area, do not feel compelled to work on every single goal every day. If you have three goals for the child in the area of communication, you may choose to focus on one of those goals each day, rotating the tasks. You will incorporate the chosen goals into the child's program all day each day.

Setting appropriate goals is important to the child's success. Observe what the child is able to do at this point, either through formal testing or by observing him. Think about the next logical step in development of that skill and set goals accordingly. By seeing what the child is able to do at this time you can figure out the next small step in the progression.

Goals will be adjusted regularly, either up or down. As children progress, you will reset the goals to a higher level. Sometimes children with autism will regress or cycle in their progress. Learning seems to stop at times, while at other times it seems to spiral. This is common and to be expected in children with autism. Cycling may be caused by a variety of factors and may not be easily remedied. The good news is that during a regression, he will most likely not lose everything he has learned, but rather a portion of it. The other good news is that as he relearns it, the recovery will usually be faster than acquiring the knowledge the first time. Cycling can be a phenomena that happens regularly and often. Take heart in the fact that this pattern decreases with age in most cases. Don't take it as a failure, and don't give up on the child when this happens. Just regroup, reset the goal and move forward once more.

⚷ KEY POINTS

- Goals are your roadmap to success.
- Set goals that are aggressive but achievable.
- State goals in positive language.

Equipment

Most programs have a limited amount of money for each teacher to spend on equipment, so choose wisely. Network with other teachers to find materials that are functional and sturdy. There is a wide range of equipment available with a vast variety of prices. Talk to civic organizations who may help with purchases. Grants may be available from a variety of sources. Perhaps you can purchase equipment to share with others who have pooled resources.

When choosing equipment, safety is your paramount concern. Keep the child's size and ability in mind as you search for items that will enhance your teaching. If you are short on toys, spread the word that you are in need of good quality toys for your classroom. Often families will donate toys when their children have outgrown them.

A growing opportunity for funding for classroom supplies is the internet. Using established sites such as *GoFundMe.com* or *Kickstarter.com*, many teachers have found success in obtaining funds for materials and projects. It requires very little set up time, and no investment, so it is surely worth a try.

KEY POINTS

- Choose equipment for the size and skill level of the child.
- Share and network to stretch your budget.

Predictability

Children on the autism spectrum have a deep need for predictability. Children like to be prepared for what is coming next. It comforts them to know what is going to happen. Creating predictability gives the child a wonderful coping skill that can help him develop control over his behaviors. The goal is not to make his whole world predictable. Many times a child's resistance to an activity or to the transition is a fear of what might happen, and a fear of the unknown. Talk him through the change. For example, if it starts to snow, you cannot control this for the child. You could not have predicted this sudden little snowstorm. What you *can do* is talk him through what is happening.

As you will remember, a PrepChat© to be helpful when facing any situation. A Prepchat© is a short talk you direct toward the child to prepare him for what is coming. Use the Prepchat© to assure him of what will happen and what rules will be followed in this situation. Simplify the rules. It may comfort him to understand the rules of the situation. A Prepchat© in this situation may go as follows:

It is starting to snow outside.

When we go to the bus there will be snow on the ground.

We will walk on the snow.

The snow will be cold but it will not hurt us.

When we get on the bus we will brush the snow off our shoes.

🔑 KEY POINTS

- Children need to know what is coming next.
- A PrepChat© is a natural method of preparing a child for what is about to happen.

Scheduling

Some tools in your bag of tricks are easy to implement, yet have a profound positive effect. Scheduling simplifies your day and keeps things on track. Posting a child friendly schedule increases the children's success. The schedule does not need to be written in words or sentences. It can certainly be a visual schedule with pictures of the daily activities. It is helpful to allow the children to move the pictures from one designation to another to indicate which activities have been completed. This is how they learn to follow the progression of the day. An individual schedule can take many different forms. Some teachers find tiny objects such as a miniature toilet, school bus, and food, which they arrange on a shelf to show order of the events of the day.

This schedule helps a child through a therapy session. He puts the check marks up as the activities are completed.

Things happen that require deviation from the schedule. Don't ignore that change in the order of events; talk them through those unexpected happenings. While predictability is important to the day to day functioning, this must be balanced with learning to cope with schedule changes. Your explanation and reassurance are important to making this adjustment.

SPEECH THERAPY		
OBJECTIVES:	SPEECH GOALS	LANGUAGE GOALS
ACTIVITY:	Self-feeding/oral motor	descriptive words during play
FINISH:	✓	✓

Many of the behavior issues in the classroom stem from problems in transitioning from one activity to another. This is particularly true when working with children who have autism. Difficulty in transitioning is one of the main identifiers of autism. You can help the children through the challenge of transitioning by providing scheduling and predictability for him. Tell him what is going to happen next. Assure him that you are there to take care of a problem if it should arise. An example of this would be to tell him that it is time to go home, but it is raining out. Tell him you will walk each child to the bus with your umbrella. Assure him that his mother will help him get dry when he gets off the bus. Remind him that he likes to ride on the bus and the bus driver is his friend. Assure him that the bus driver and the bus monitor will take care of him on the bus, even when it is raining.

Sebastian was fully potty trained at home. When he entered preschool, he reverted to soiling his pants daily. Even though the teachers encouraged him sporadically throughout the day to use the restroom, (especially when they saw signs that an accident might be imminent) toileting was not on a strict schedule for the class. He struggled with transition of any type, and could not embrace the concept of stopping his play to go to the bathroom as needed. Teachers used visual timers to allow Sebastian to accept the transition to potty time more easily.

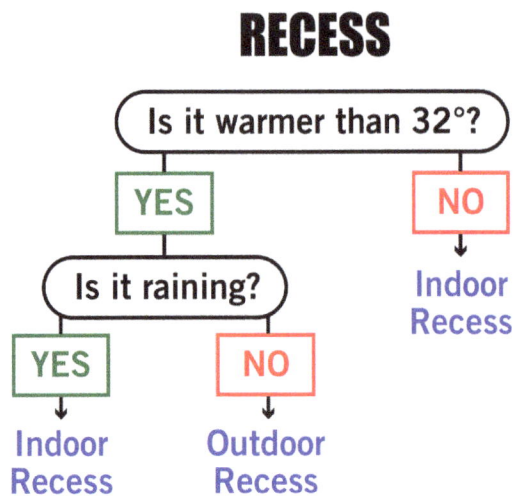

RECESS

Is it warmer than 32°?

YES — Is it raining?

YES — Indoor Recess

NO — Outdoor Recess

NO — Indoor Recess

Here is an idea for older children who can read, which saves a lot of teacher time in answering that all-important question, "Are we going outside today?"

Another tip for aiding in transition is to tell them the plan for ending the activity as you start it. As he is getting on the bus to go home, remind him that when the bus gets to his house, he will get off. If the children are on the way to the lunchroom, remind them that when lunch is over, Miss Kelly will bring them back to the play area. When you start an activity let them know when it will be over and what will happen to them at that point.

Setting a timer for the activity is helpful. You can obtain visual timers that are very effective with this population. Give a countdown to aid in transition. Announce that we will be putting the toys away in two minutes. Add another reminder at the one-minute mark, then a quick countdown at the very end of the activity, "Three, two, one. Time to put the books on the shelf." If the child is still not transitioning well, you may have to be more direct. Gently help the child comply if he will not do it unaided. This does not mean forcing or being aggressive. The child is likely not being directly disobedient, but having true difficulty in removing himself from the current activity. For children with special challenges, transitioning can be an emotional time, so don't take it personally.

🔑 KEY POINTS

• Scheduling simplifies your task and provides predictability for the children.
• When you begin a task give information about the ending of the task.
• Visual schedules are an effective teaching tool.

Coping Strategies

Another critical tool in your bag of tricks consists of a gift that the teacher will give to the child. This is the gift of a set of coping skills that will serve him for the rest of his life. When you teach him strategies for coping with unexpected or unpleasant situation, you have given him a tool to gain control over his own behavior. This, in turn, becomes a gift he gives to you. If the adults in a child's life do not teach him positive coping skills, he will resort to coping skills which may not be socially acceptable, such as tantrums, withdrawal, or acting out. A child who can learn to calm himself has a tool for life. When a child can employ a calming coping skill he remains more ready to learn.

Dustin was a child on the autism spectrum who struggled with obsessive compulsive disorder and a great deal of anxiety. He became anxious when seeing a spider in the room, during thunderstorms, and when hearing sirens in the distance, among other triggers. Dustin's obsessive compulsive tendencies extended to others also. He would get very frustrated when other people did things the "wrong" way. Dustin's teacher worked with him to help him learn to recognize the pounding heart, the shortness of breath and the sweaty palms that signaled the beginnings of anxiety and frustration. She was also very careful to observe specific situations that she knew would be hard for Dustin to handle so she could be pro-active in her support of his emerging coping skills. Dustin's teacher hit upon the idea of having him take deep, calming breaths as he repeated to himself, "It's no biggie! It's no biggie!" With the teacher supporting him and reminding him how and when to breathe slowly and repeat his mantra, Dustin gained a tool he could use independently anywhere, any time his anxiety and frustration with others became too much for him. This allowed Dustin to spend more time with his peers, in new situations, and in public places.

Sometimes visual supports can be helpful as calming tools as well. The child needs to be taught how to look at the visual to help himself calm, and will need to practice how that works with you, probably multiple times. This visual can help a child express their level of frustration or anger, and work toward calming.

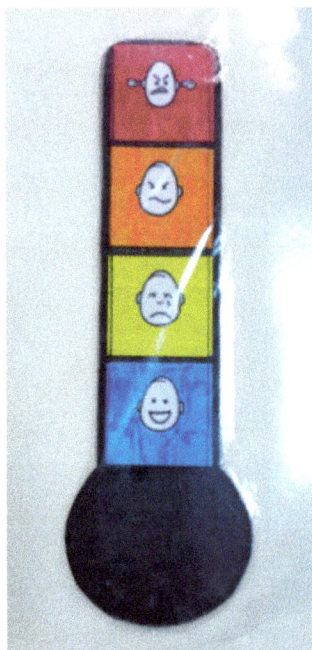

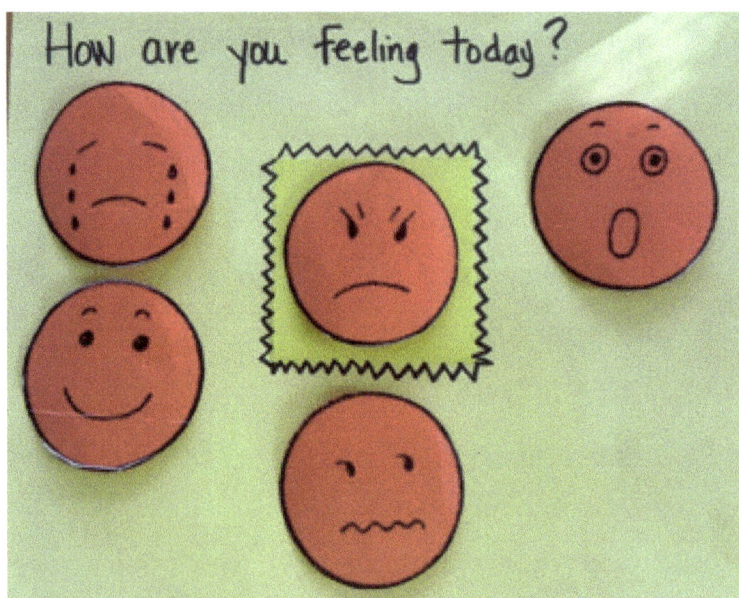

A child who has not learned socially appropriate coping skills will develop and exhibit his own. These may be not only socially inappropriate, such as screaming or kicking, they may actually be harmful to the child, such as biting himself. We have seen children who have developed large red calluses on their hands from biting themselves in an effort to calm down. They may exhibit this activity when there is stress or when they are happily excited. They must learn coping strategies to cope with the positive as well as the negative energy they encounter.

🔑 KEY POINTS

- There are coping skills that are positive and coping skills that are negative.
- Teach strategies for positive coping skills.
- If children are not taught acceptable coping skills, they will develop inappropriate ways of coping.

Task Analysis

When you are teaching a skill, especially to children with special needs, your success is dependent on your ability to break down the task into smaller, simpler steps. The process you will rely on for this is known as. When you start using this technique to teach, you will be surprised at the tiny steps that make up an action. Good task analysis serves multiple purposes. [19] It provides you with baby steps that the child can attain much more successfully than mastering a complex task all at once. Breaking down the action into small steps lets you and the child see success earlier. Celebrate success at every step as it is attained. If you have a goal on the IEP that is not being met, take a step back and break it down even further. Task analysis is most often successful when working with children who have a difficult time remembering and following complex directions, such as children with ADHD, autism, or those who are cognitively challenged.

Tasks are broken down to the level that each child can understand and complete. You might break down the task of washing his face into twenty small steps. If needed, each of those steps could easily be broken down even further. For example, if you are working on the step, "picking up the washcloth," that requires the behaviors of locating the washcloth, reaching toward it, grasping it, turning the cloth toward the face, etc. How small you decide to make the steps will depend on your child's ability to follow the sequential steps. While some children would need twenty increments in order to become competent in that action, others may grasp it when taught in five steps.

Here is an example of a task analysis for washing his face:

1. Come into the bathroom
2. Get the little stool
3. Bring the stool to the sink
4. Stand on the stool
5. Grab the washcloth
6. Turn on the water
7. Wet the washcloth
8. Rub soap on the washcloth
9. Touch the cloth to your face
10. Move the cloth around the face
11. Put the cloth down
12. Cup hands in the flow of water
13. Close your eyes
14. Splash water on face to rinse
15. Open eyes
16. Pick up washcloth
17. Move washcloth to the sink
18. Rinse out washcloth
19. Wring water out of washcloth
20. Hang up washcloth to dry

As you progress through the list of behaviors that make up a task, also known as **chaining**, you might start with the first step on the list, such as, "pick up the washcloth." You may use a hand-over-hand technique to teach that step. As he becomes successful with that increment, you add step two, "move it to the sink", etc.

An alternative method which you will prefer in some cases is to teach the task from the last step backward to the first step. In other words, complete the task for the child while you talk aloud about each thing you are doing. When you get to the last step, "Hang up the washcloth to dry," let the child complete that final step. When he has mastered that, add the second to last step, which may be "wring out the washcloth." Using this technique, you are in essence, backward chaining. Another example of backward chaining that many people find successful is in teaching a child to tie his shoes. You may demonstrate the chain of events tying the shoe as you talk about what you are doing. When you come to the final, "Pull both loops," you turn the task over to the child and he finishes the job. As he masters that task, it gives him a sense of accomplishment and pride. The next time you add the second to last step to what he performs and with your coaching he will do those last two steps. You will build on this step by step in this backward direction until he can do all of the steps either independently or with prompting, depending on your IEP goal. Students who have cognitive, physical or communication impairments can benefit from this process, just as a typical learner can.

If the child is having difficulty attaining any of the steps, break that step down even further into smaller steps. Analyze each task and think about ways to allow the child to enjoy the success of achieving goals through baby steps.

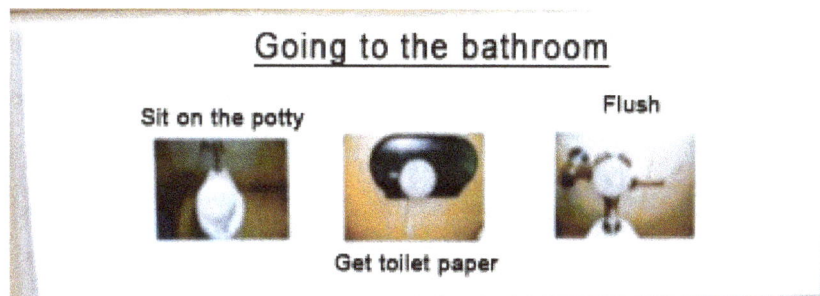

Going to the bathroom

Sit on the potty

Flush

Get toilet paper

When it comes time for teachers to give parents a quarterly progress report, you will certainly have some good news to include on the report if you have been diligent in breaking the task into small steps. While a goal of, "Washes his hands independently" might result in a report of "Not mastered," you will have more positive news when you tell the parent that the child has now learned to, "Climb onto the stepstool," "Turn on the water," and "Pick up the soap. He has mastered, "Rubbing the soap onto his hands." You may then explain that you will continue to support him in this goal by teaching him the next step of, "Rinsing off the soap," "Turning off the water," and "Drying his hands."

A checklist is a handy tool that helps a child as he learns to sequence the tasks. Allow him to check off each segments as he performs the job, this will clue him to independently learn what step comes next.

🔑 KEY POINTS

- Break any task into its smaller parts.
- Teach the sequence of a task from either the first step or the last step.
- If the child is having significant difficulty mastering any given step, break that one down even further.

Visual Supports

Visual prompts and visual aids make very effective teaching tools. A picture really is worth a thousand words, especially when teaching children with autism, those with developmental delays, language processing issues and challenging behaviors.

The main challenges for a child with autism are social interactions and using language appropriately. Visual supports can help with those challenges.

Visuals can:

- help a student focus
- make an abstract concept more concrete
- help a child express thoughts or feelings
- reduce anxiety
- provide routine, structure and a sequence of activities
- help with transitions

Visuals can help teach social skills such as simple greetings or how to start a conversation. They can help to "translate" spoken instructions from an adult. Visual cues may help a child begin to communicate very abstract information such as feelings. These supports can help children understand the sequence of activities in their day, which can reduce anxiety. The uses of visuals in the classroom are almost endless. You will want to make your visual as interactive as possible. Using Velcro™ on the backs of your pictures will allow the child to move the picture themselves or to hand it to an adult to request an item. Just like any new skills, you will need to spend a certain amount of time with your student to teach the how to use the visual. The possibilities are endless, but here are some examples to think about.

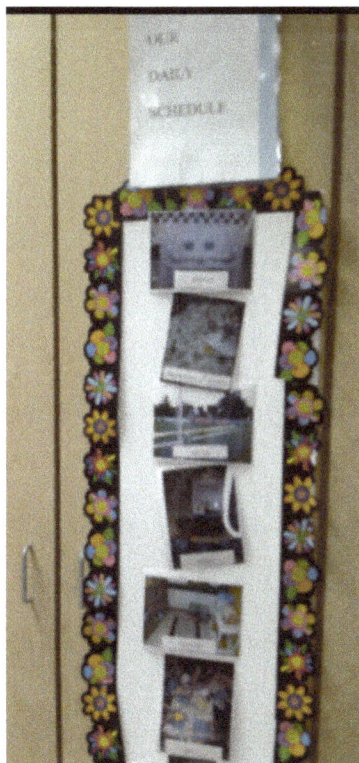

Here is a picture schedule similar to those introduced earlier. It shows the sequence of the day's activities for the class. This is helpful for all the children in your classroom, but will really benefit those on the spectrum. Pictures can be made with Velcro™ on them so the sequence can be changed as needed. You may want to indicate the current activity with a moveable arrow, clothespin or marker. If you consistently use this each day in the classroom as you talk with your students at circle time or morning meeting, your students will begin to use this as a reference during the day just as you use your day planner. The schedule can be either horizontal or vertical, but be sure you move either left to right (the same direction you read) or from top to bottom. Children with high anxiety or a real need to know what's next can benefit by helping you move the arrow.

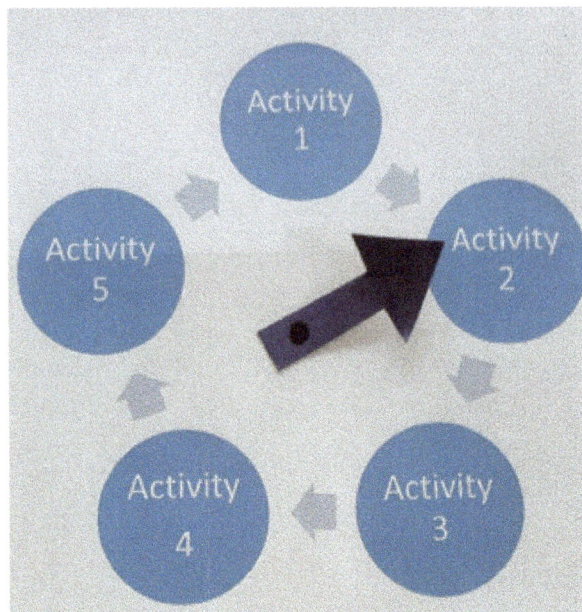

This can be used as either a schedule for an entire class or exclusively for an individual student. There are many pictures online that can be downloaded, but many students respond best to real pictures of their very own classroom.

Other helpful examples can found with the commercially available program called PECS®, or Picture Exchange Communication System©.[13] This system could help a child communicate feelings or needs that might otherwise be difficult to communicate. When a visual is first put into place, it's important to work with the child to assure he understands how to use it, and what it can communicate. Be sure the visual support is not too complicated for the child. For a very young child, you may want to simplify this to just two or three pictures. PECS® is used following formal training by the teacher.

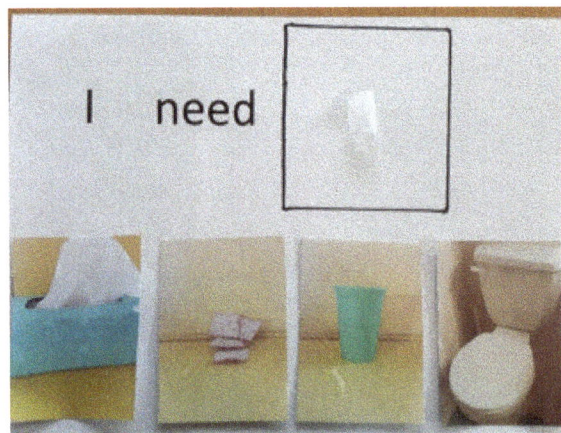

Here is another example in which the child is able to choose what they need and communicate this message by sticking the appropriate picture in the sentence strip. For young children, it's most effective if they can interact with the visual system by moving a picture themselves. This gives them a sense of power and ownership.

First-then charts can help students complete a non-preferred task before a preferred chore. The preferred task becomes the reward. Children can easily see how many things are left on their "to-do" list.

The first-then chart allows the adult to sequence activities and is useful for requesting the child to complete a non-preferred activity before a preferred one, and to follow directions. As you teach a child to use a first-then visual, start with preferred and familiar activities until the child is competent at using the new visual.

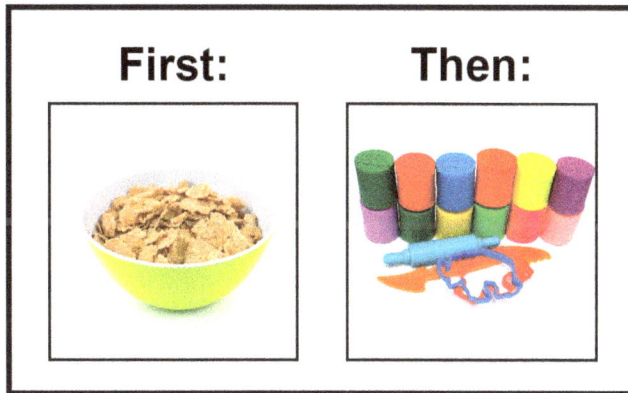

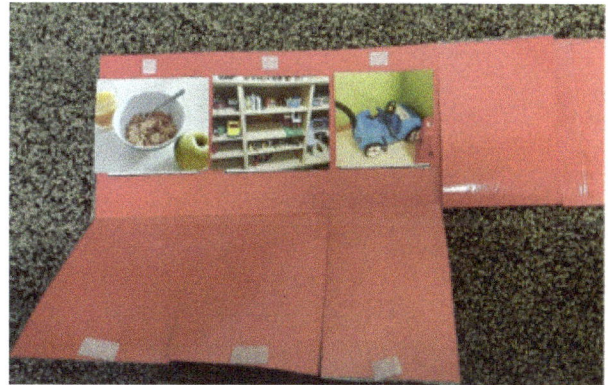

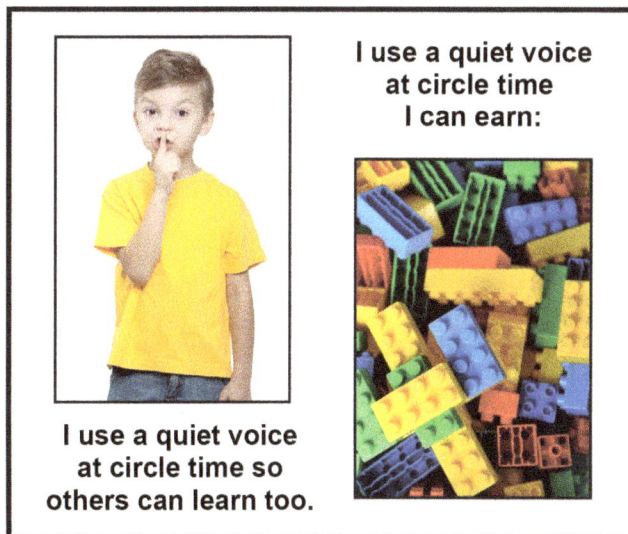

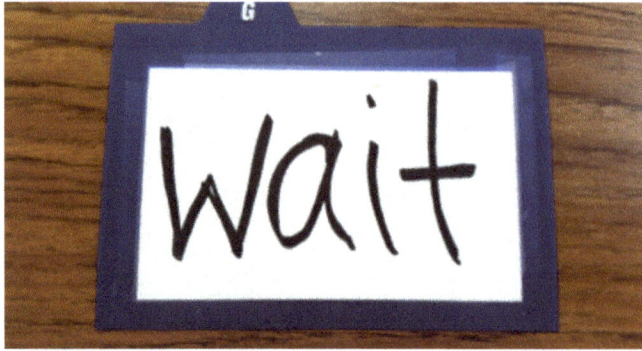

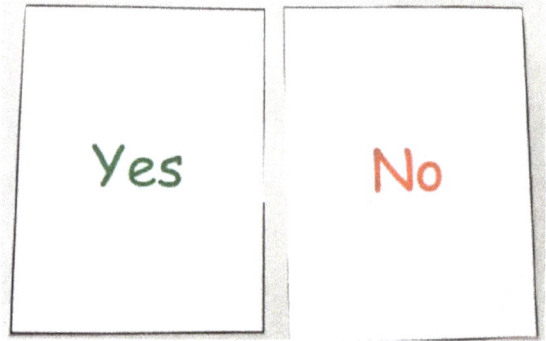

Waiting can be hard, but this visual served as an effective reminder for a little one who had trouble waiting in line for even a few seconds. He had the visual of the word and had the sensory experience of holding the reminder in his hand.

Learning to teach by the use of a visual is a new skill for the teacher; you will need to devote some time to teaching the child to use it. Be sure to use it consistently and to introduce it each time with some verbal cue such as, "Let's check your schedule" or "Let's use your work chart" etc.

Rewards and Reinforcers

A reward or a reinforcer is something that is greatly preferred by the child, not by you. It can be time with a special person, a sensory activity, or a favorite toy. Think outside the box! Just because it's not rewarding to you, doesn't mean it's not rewarding to them. For students on the spectrum who are very linear and concrete thinkers that take you at your word, you must be sure to follow through with the promised reinforcer; otherwise, you have lost all credibility with the child. Even with a very preferred reinforcer, a child will eventually

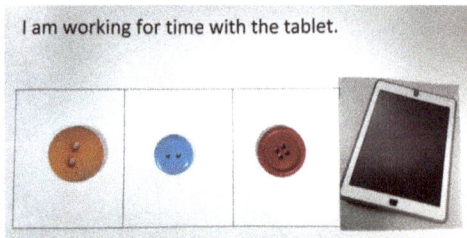

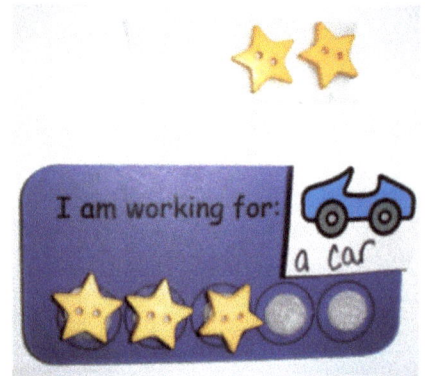

124

satiate, or get tired of the reinforcer, indicating that it is time for a new motivator.

Observing what your child really likes in the classroom, or talking with parents will give you some good ideas. For more visual ideas than you can possibly use in this lifetime, check Pinterest.com or do a web search. Good terms to search for are "visual schedules" or "visual supports for autism." You can check for ideas, apps and computer programs to help you. As always, some apps will be free, some will cost, and new ones are continually being developed.

www.autismspeaks.org
www.livingwellwithautism.com
www.schKIDules.com
www.autismparentingmagazine.com
https://autoplaytherapy.com/resources//

Parents and therapists can direct you to specific resources that have been helpful to them, so be sure to ask.

🔑 KEY POINTS

- Visual supports can help with transitions and clarify expectations.
- Learning to use the visual support is a new skill that may take time to learn.

Peer Helpers

A powerful tool in working with students who have any type of special need is the enlistment of peer helpers. Children are usually very altruistic by nature; they like to do the right thing. You will have students in your classroom who will benefit from the opportunity to help and teach others as well. Peers can be invited into almost any situation in which a child needs to practice turn taking, social greetings, conversation or play skills. The potential for interactions is endless.

Observing all of your children at play will give you a very good idea of which child will make a great peer helper in a given setting. Make sure to tell the peer helper what your goal is for the other child; he needs to be in on the game. It's appropriate to say, "Jasmine is learning how to play in the kitchen. Would you like to join us and show her how we use the utensils?" This is a great way to build community within the classroom- we all help each other. Do be sure to use your peers wisely. Don't always rely on the same helper. You want the situation to be enjoyable for them as well. Just as with adults, some children mesh better with others, regardless of disability, so keep personalities in mind too. A very shy child may be overwhelmed by a very confident one, or may really enjoy the interaction, so give it a try and see how it goes. Do make sure your peer helpers know that your special needs students have strengths as well as things they are learning. It's easy to fall into the trap of inadvertently allowing a peer helper to think he already knows everything, but he doesn't! That's a learning opportunity for the helpers.

One example of a peer really stepping up was the interaction between Sheridan and Kandace. Sheridan was a nonverbal child with multiple disabilities who was learning to use pictures to make requests at snack time. She had been working with the teacher and speech therapist on this task successfully for several weeks. She would hand the adult the picture of the snack she wanted, the adult would provide the snack bite and replace the picture on a Velcro™ board so she could repeat the request. Kandace, a very confident young lady, had some behavior issues. She happened to be sitting by Sheridan one day and asked if she could give her the snack. The teacher thought it was worth a try and was stunned at how well Kandace had learned the specific picture/snack routine and how well Sheridan responded to getting a snack from a peer. Success! It was a great opportunity for Kandace to get some recognition for being an expert at something.

Pets Are Positive

You may consider using pets in your classroom. Pets teach children responsibility and empathy while providing non-judgmental companionship that may be less intimidating than human company. Another great option is pet therapy, if you have that available in your community. A volunteer can visit your class and bring an animal, usually dog, cat or rabbit. All animals that are part of a pet therapy program have to pass rigorous testing in order to ensure a pleasant temperament and the willingness to be handled. Sometimes the animals are trained to do tricks, and the owners are usually very friendly, engaging visitors. Nonverbal children can be encouraged to use words to give the pet directions or praise. Watching the animal respond to their commands or gestures or even approach the child for a treat, can be incredibly empowering and confidence-building in a young child. Learning to interact appropriately with an animal can pave the way for more appropriate human interactions. Of course, make sure that no child in your class has an allergy to the animals before the event or before adding a pet to the classroom. It's always a good idea to check with all the parents in your classroom to see if any of your students have any particular fears related to animals. That is not a reason to preclude animals from visiting, but gives you, as teacher, an idea of how best to introduce the visitor to make it stress-free for everyone. It sometimes happens that those children who are initially fearful of animals are the ones who end up loving the pets the most- it just takes an appropriate introduction to the situation. An online search or a call to a local veterinarian's office can put you in touch with someone from a local pet therapy organization.

Chapter 8

SOS! Sharing our Strategies

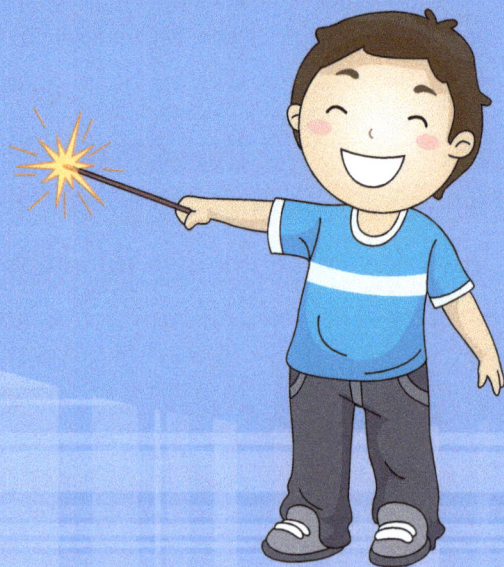

Strategies to Address Elopement

A major concern when working with children with ASD is the danger of them eloping or wandering away. Elope simply means to run off. While some children with autism tend to just wander away, others are runners. Runners have a strong desire to escape from their environment. These children sometimes have a plan in mind, however misguided it may be. Perhaps they are continually trying to leave because they think they can get to a store for candy. Maybe they want to go to Disneyland and see Mickey Mouse. Others run off because they actually enjoy having you chase them. To them, this is a fun game. As they run, they will look back immediately to see if you are chasing them, and laugh as they see you running after them.

Before you can determine how you will handle this running behavior, you have to stop and think about which of these categories he falls into. Is he trying to get to a destination or is he looking for a fun game of chase? Door alarms are often a helpful preventative for runners. If you have a runner or a wanderer, put alarms on as many of the barrier doors as possible, including fences. While these kids are talented little Houdinis and expert escape artists, the alarms and multiple locks and security codes can at least slow them down. Be very firm with the parents that they should not allow the children to push the door releases or the door codes as they leave the school. These should be strictly for the use of adults only.

KEY POINTS

- If a child is wandering or running from the class you will need to determine the reason he is doing this before you can address the behavior.
- Safety is a primary concern in any classroom.

Strategies for Reducing Aggression

Aggression is the extreme end of social adjustment. There are different types of aggression, with different motivations. One child may be only aggressive toward adults, while another is only aggressive toward other children, and yet a third may direct his anger toward inanimate objects. Aggression must be handled in a manner consistent with the other team members. It must be addressed early before it becomes a firmly ingrained habit for the child. We need to give him other ways to express his anger before it escalates to a dangerous level. If the object of his aggression is other children, every precaution must be taken to keep the other children safe. This is your priority.

Children who attack adults in the environment but are not aggressive toward other children have sometimes learned that while another child may return the physical assault, the adults will not. They have figured out that if they hit the teacher, the teacher will not hit back. If they kick the teacher or spit on the teacher, the teacher cannot return the action. Aggression must be addressed within the child's IEP or the Behavior Intervention Plan (BIP). The team will decide what consequences are meaningful to this particular child, and all caregivers must be consistent. Behavior Intervention Plans are legal documents that are created with the agreement of the teacher, parent, and other team professionals. BIPs address the target behavior and the strategies that the team agrees to use to address those behaviors. It is often a reward-based system. The plan should be used consistently by all caregivers and service providers.

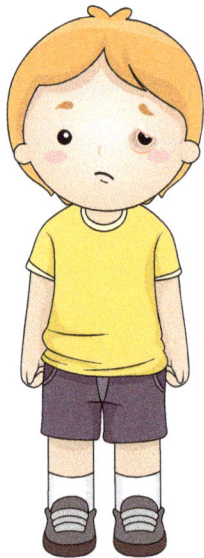

The team will need to think about the child's motivation in the aggression. Is it attention seeking, or is it born of frustration at not being able to communicate? Is the child trying to get something or to escape something? Being a good observer of when the behavior occurs and what happens afterwards will help you decode the

130

motivation. Along with identifying the usual object of the aggression, you will need to determine whether the behavior is attention seeking. If it seems to be driven by a need for attention, your plan will be to give a consequence that eliminates attention, rather than gives any type of attention. This consequence may include removing him to a less stimulating room or area. When he displays positive, non-aggressive behaviors, *that* is the time to give him the attention he craves.

Aggressive behavior may be a mechanism the child learns as an escape behavior. You can teach the child more acceptable coping methods when a situation gets overwhelming for him. Help the child find ways to calm himself and find other outlets for the anxiety he is feeling. Sometimes a small tactile activity such as silly putty can offer just enough stimulation and distraction to allow the child to make it through a difficult situation without getting aggressive. Headphones work in many noisy environments to prevent the meltdown that can lead to aggressive outbursts.

If attention does not seem to be his main motive for the aggression, you will need to observe him to determine what sets off the behavior. Aggressive behaviors can be modified.

🔑 KEY POINTS

- There are various causes for aggression and a teacher can figure out what causes aggression in a specific situation.
- Aggression must be addressed before it becomes a firmly established habit.
- Teach children methods to calm themselves.

Strategies to Reduce Random Verbalizations

Some children with autism make random noises all day. They may make humming noises, they may mutter to themselves, or they may yell out. Sometimes they sound like they are chanting. This is another area where you will need to be a detective and figure out the motivation of the child for the vocalizations.

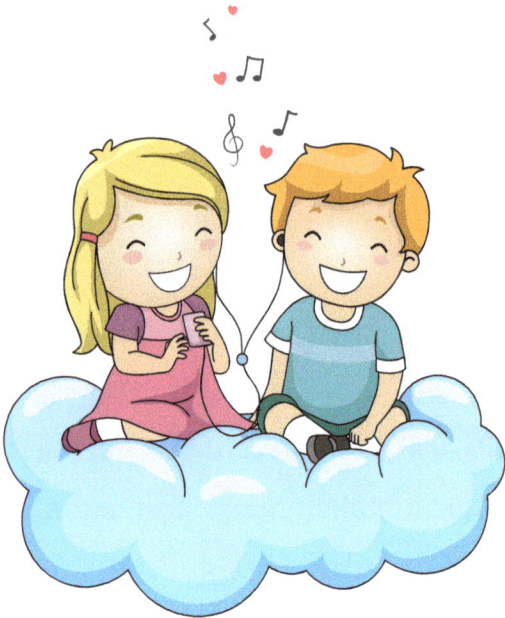

Some children do chanting or humming noises constantly to block out other noises in their environment that may be irritating to them. They could be trying to mask a noise as minimal as the buzzing in the lights or the fan in the air conditioning. These children are highly sensitive to noises and are trying to block them out. Some people have found it helpful to offer children the use of noise reducing headphones if they produce continual random verbalizations.

Other children may shout out randomly to gain attention. If you think the behavior is attention seeking, once again, the consequence must to remove him from attention, not to shower him with attention.

Still other children may make random vocalizations as a way of self-stimulating. You may give him an alternate, less disruptive, stimulating activity, such as gum to chew or a Cush™ ball to hold.

🔑 KEY POINTS

- Children may make random noises to filter out noises or voices in the environment.
- If a child shouts out to gain attention, do not reinforce that behavior by giving him the attention he is seeking.

Strategies to Reduce Self-Injurious Behaviors

You may have a child in your class who seems to be trying to mutilate himself. Perhaps he bites his arm, or pulls out his hair, or picks at mosquito bites until they are open sores the size of half dollars. This is yet another case where you need to look at the child's motivation. He may be

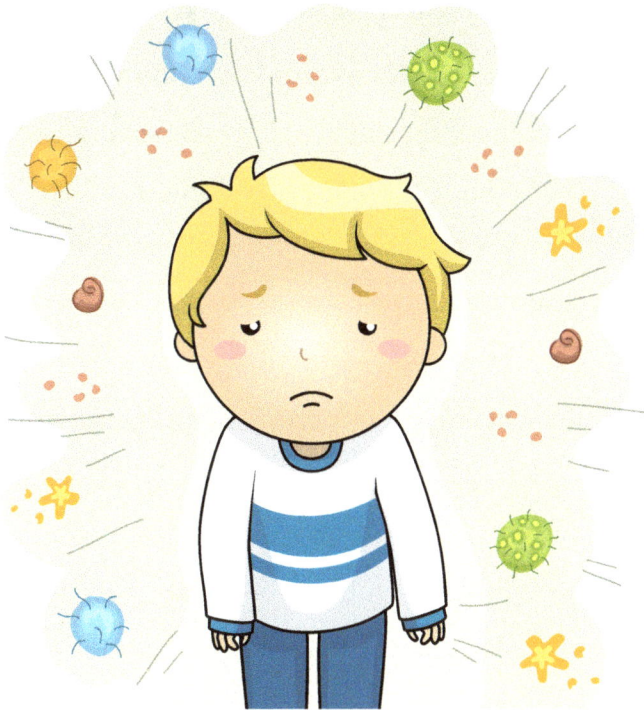

fulfilling a sensory need, he might do this as a ritualistic behavior, he could be misinterpreting stimuli, or it may be comforting to them. A child may bite his hand to attempt to calm himself when he is overly excited at play. While there are emotionally disturbed children who are truly self-destructive, the children we describe here seldom fit into that category. Like most behaviors of autism, if we can understand the cause of the behavior we can help the child develop a strategy to eliminate it. Most of these children are using the behavior to meet some need, either sensory or calming.

As most children with autism are stringent rule followers, a strategy you can use is to tell them there is a rule against this behavior. With constant reminding they may replace that behavior with something more acceptable. The key here is to give them a replacement behavior. Don't just expect them to eliminate an action without giving them an alternate behavior.

🔑 KEY POINTS

- If a child appears to be hurting himself on purpose you will need to figure out his motivation.
- This may be an attempt to calm himself.
- He may be trying to meet a sensory need.
- Rather than trying to simply eliminate the behavior, give them a replacement activity.

Strategies to Reduce Aggression or Distress in Response to Noise

Sometime children are overly sensitive to noise and they try to avoid that stimuli. Children may cry, scream, or become upset when the environment becomes noisy. This is especially true of sudden sounds. The reaction may be brought on as noise volumes increase. For some this may happen in response to only certain sounds -- such as voices. The child may react by covering his ears or hiding under the table or chairs. High pitched sounds may be particularly troublesome to this group. Metallic sounds may irritate him. Behaviors may include avoiding the sound of toilets flushing, water flowing, or electric hand dryers.

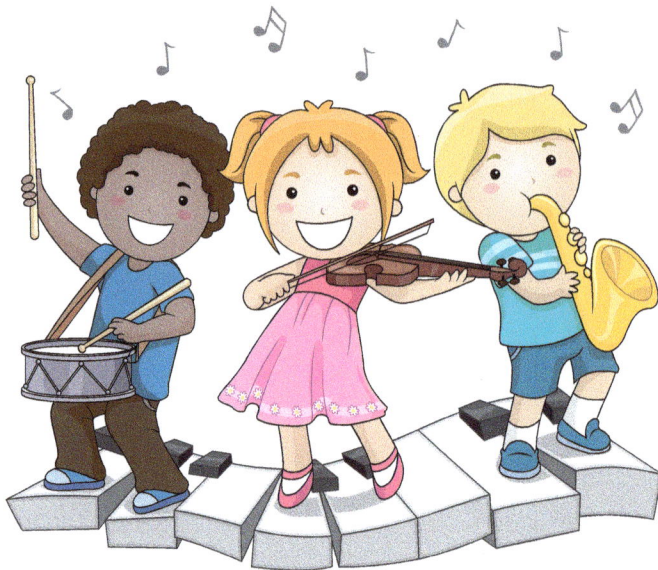

There is a difference between what a child physically *hears* and what his brain perceives. **Auditory processing** is the means by which the brain processes sounds into meaningful information. Some children can *hear* perfectly well, but have difficulty processing that information. It is difficult for them to make sense out of complex sounds, such as speech, especially when there is a noisy background. They have difficulty listening to two speakers at the same time.

Being a detective is not always easy. Things aren't always what they seem. A grandma took her granddaughter into the restroom at church. The little girl dutifully put her hands over her ears as she entered, and kept them there the entire time as Grandma helped her on and off the potty. Only when it was time to wash her hands did Katie take her hands off her ears. Grandma reported back to Katie's mom that Katie must really hate the sound of the toilets and hand dryers because she had covered her ears with her hands. Mom explained that in reality, she had simply taught Katie the habit of putting her hands on her ears to eliminate the chance of her touching anything in the restrooms.

Other children may exhibit behaviors in response to being hyposensitive to sounds. They seek out sounds to fill this need. They prefer loud music. They talk loudly, seeming always to shout. When given a musical instrument or other noise producing instrument they hold it close to their ears. The seem to crave noises, and may sit and listen to fans or water running for a long period of time.

Activities which may help children with auditory sensitivities will depend on whether the child is hypo or hypersensitive. Helpful interventions include the use of headphones or earplugs, having a quiet space available where the child can get away from the noise, and listen to calming music. Sound machines may be effective in masking out noise. Other kids may do well with games that require close listening, such as matching sounds, singing, rhymes, and chants, or musical instruments. They like to listen to pre-recorded books. Pay attention to what the need seems to be, either auditory seeking or auditory avoiding, and feed that need.

KEY POINTS

- Sounds, sights, or touches in the environment may result in unwanted behaviors.
- Determine if the behavior is sensory avoiding or sensory seeking.
- There is a difference between what the brain hears and what the brain perceives.

Strategies to Reduce Unwanted Behaviors in Response to Visual Stimuli

Some behaviors that children exhibit may be attempts to avoid light because they are too sensitive to it. This may be obvious, such as a child avoiding bright lights and sunlight. covering the eyes or squinting or attempting to screen out light using a variety of methods.

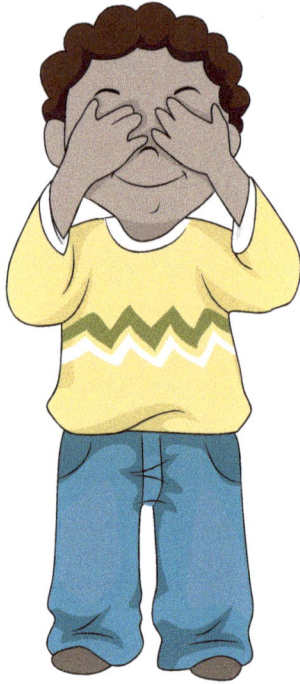

Sensitivity to light may be less obvious, such as a child who is afraid of moving objects, has frequent headaches or dizziness. He may rub his eyes a lot, or seem unable to judge distance. He may seem clumsy as he is unaware of objects in his path. He may not be able to determine contrasting colors well. Light cozies are rectangular pieces of cloth that attach over the fluorescent lights on the ceiling to soften the glare. These easy to install products are commercially available. We do not recommend that you make your own, due to possible fire hazards.

On the other hand, some children actually seek out visual stimuli. They may even go so far as to stare at a flashlight. They enjoy bright lights and direct sunlight. You may see them move or shake their heads during seat work. They may enjoy looking closely at an object as if they are examining it. They may not seem to even notice people or objects around them. They have difficulty focusing on objects, and frequently lose their place when looking at a page. They like visually stimulating patterns.

As with the auditory activities, you will need to determine whether the child is seeking or avoiding the visual stimuli, then present activities to meet that need. He may benefit from visual schedules, or by reducing clutter in the room. Give frequent "eye breaks." Try color matching games or games that require keeping the eye on a target. Flashlight tag is fun, especially with little pen lights. If you have a light table, that may be effective. Art activities that include drawing, painting, cutting on a line or gluing are helpful. If a child can do mazes or labyrinths, these may help sustain visual attention. Children of many ages can play "I spy" and learn to scan the room visually.

🔑 KEY POINTS

- Children who cover their eyes or squint may be attempting to block out light that is overwhelming to them.
- Children with light sensitivities may be afraid of moving objects.
- Children with light sensitivities may not discriminate colors well.
- Some children may seek visual stimulation.
- Children who are seeking visual stimuli may benefit from an uncluttered environment and visual schedules.

Strategies to Reduce Unwanted Behaviors in Response to Touch or Feeling

Some behavior problems are due to hypersensitivity to touch. These children may try to avoid certain textures or some items of clothing (or *all* clothing, in some cases). Tight pants, scratchy tags, seams and new materials cause distress. These children do not enjoy muddy or messy play. They don't like dirty hands or hands covered with paint or other art supplies. This is complicated by the fact that they do not like hand or face washing, either. They are more ticklish that the average child, and often avoid hugs or other physical contact. Light touch is almost painful. They usually fuss about hair washing, hair brushing, or combing. These kids are often fussy eaters due to not liking the textures of the food. They may not like the feel of going barefoot, and sometimes tend to "toe walk."

Three-year-old Marie is on the autism spectrum and is very sensory avoiding. Her avoidance takes the form of aversion to any

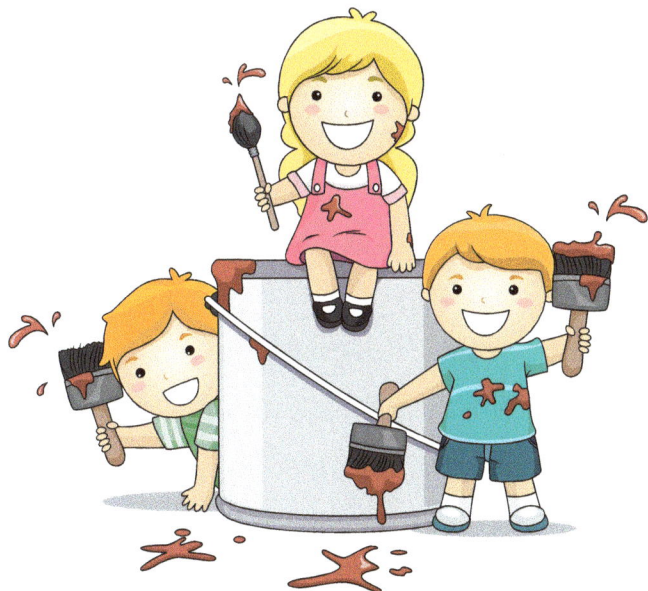

sticky, slick or slimy texture in projects and play. We could say that Marie is *tactile defensive*. Marie's teacher gave up "making her" participate in sensory play just like everybody else. Instead, she allowed Marie some simple accommodations, such as allowing Marie to wear an old pair of gloves for finger painting, allowing her some toys to play with in the shaving cream, which made it far more appealing, and allowing her to spread glue with a Q tip rather than her finger. The teacher allows Marie to use a wet wipe on her hands right after playing with Play-Doh®, and knowing she can clean her hands quickly has made Marie more willing to touch and manipulate Play-Doh®. Sensory activities are no longer a power struggle, and the teacher rightly anticipates that as Marie gets older, she will be less concerned about these sensitivities.

The flip side of this are the children who are striving to increase their tactile input. These kids prefer tight clothing, and often dress in layers to achieve that feeling of pressure. They are often dirty or messy as they are drawn to those situations. They are not usually aware that they are being touched by others, and have a high pain tolerance. Low impulse control gets them into trouble, as they like to touch everything and often hurt other children. They often hit, push and pinch others. They crave vibration. They dislike hair brushing, or hair washing, they may crave certain strong flavors and constantly mouth inedible objects.

While some children are driven to avoid certain sensations, others crave those stimuli. Greg was, as his parents said, "wound tight." He was always busy, never sitting still, was very creative in his play and loved to learn. However, Greg had trouble focusing in his preschool classroom. His teacher talked a lot with parents about "getting ready" for kindergarten, and used daily worksheets. Sitting at a table for a prolonged time, coloring in shapes and cutting them out didn't teach Greg much. It made it very difficult to meet the need he had for movement. This resulted in behavior issues and power struggles with the very traditional teacher. Once the teacher began to see that Greg's misbehavior was always related to table time, she began to examine her own teaching practices more closely. She changed some of the learning activities in the classroom, and made them more child-friendly, incorporating movement and whole body experiences. For example, instead of having to color a letter of the alphabet, the children began to use Play-Doh® to make the letter, finger paint the letter, play a letter/beanbag game, participate in music and movement games to learn the letter, and do a letter search around the room. This helped not only Greg, but many of the children, to focus and participate better. They became more actively engaged in their learning and were able to retain more of what they learned. In addition, the teacher now understands Greg's needs better and can allow him some extra activity when he needs it. The teacher keeps a box filled with several unopened reams of paper that Greg can pull around the room with a jump rope handle when he feels the need for some activity. This "heavy work" actually helps Greg to expend energy and calm himself down. On rainy days, the teacher now brings a mini-trampoline into the room, and incorporates additional movement activities during music time. She is aware now of the strong connection between the mind and the body and that young children are wired to move as they learn. Changing her teaching style combined with meeting Greg's individual needs has resulted in huge positive changes in the classroom.

To help these children work through those behaviors, once again, watch to determine whether the child is seeking tactile sensations or avoiding them. Some suggested tactile activities include filling bins with rice, flour, beans, etc. to create sensory bins. You may hide small objects in the bin and let him dig through the materials to find treasure. Make various dough textures using recipes found on the internet. Finger painting is a good activity for those seeking tactile sensation. These kids may enjoy a massage or hand squeezes. Surround him with pillows or roll him in blankets like a burrito. Weighted vests and blankets may be comforting.

Many children who have tactile sensitivity to touch tolerate it much better when presented as a firm touch, rather than a feathery light touch. Another suggestion when working with tactile sensitive children is to verbally prepare them for the touch so that it does not send them into a tailspin. An example of this would be, "Jax, I am going to move your hand to show you how to zip this coat."

🔑 KEY POINTS

- Tactile sensations can lead to many unwanted behaviors.
- Watch to determine whether the child is seeking tactile sensations or avoiding them.
- A firm touch may be better tolerated than a light touch.
- A verbal notice before touching a child may be helpful.

Strategies to Reduce Unwanted Behaviors in Response to Body Awareness Issues

Children with difficulties in proprioception will have difficulties with body awareness. They may appear to be lazy or seem lethargic. They try to avoid physical activity, even normal playground activities. They just prefer to sit. They usually avoid touch from others and can often be a picky eater. They seem to be uncoordinated. Even when they are doing a familiar activity such as going up and down stairs, they rely on deep concentration and a visual cue.

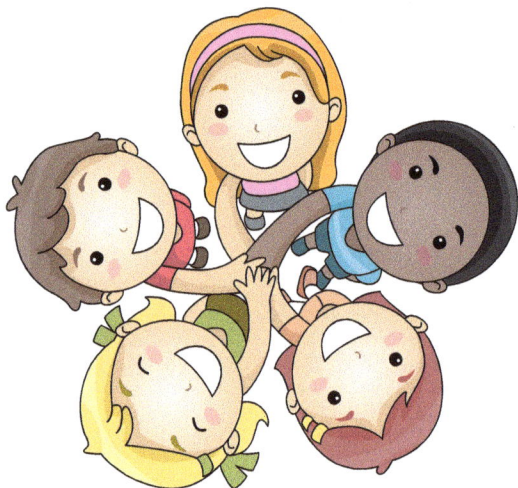

Others are seeking out that same feedback. They are the kids who often bump into walls or other people. The are forceful and they stomp around or walk loudly. They are rough as they kick, bite and hit others. They have a poor awareness of personal space. They are comforted by wearing tight clothing or layers of clothing. They like to chew on non-edible objects such as pencils, shirts, or even their fingers.

As with each of the other senses, the teacher's job is to discover whether the child is seeking or avoiding proprioceptive stimuli. Helpful activities can include firm bear hugs, massages, walking like an animal, bouncing on trampolines, doing pushups from the floor or from a wall, carrying items of appropriate weight, yoga, or playing with Play-Doh®.

🔑 KEY POINTS

- Some children avoid physical activity and others crave it.
- Children with proprioceptive issues are uncoordinated and may bump into walls or objects.
- Some children with body awareness struggles prefer to wear layers of clothing.
- They may chew on non-edible objects.
- There are sensory activities that help with this challenge.

Strategies to Avoid Behaviors Associated with Balance Problems

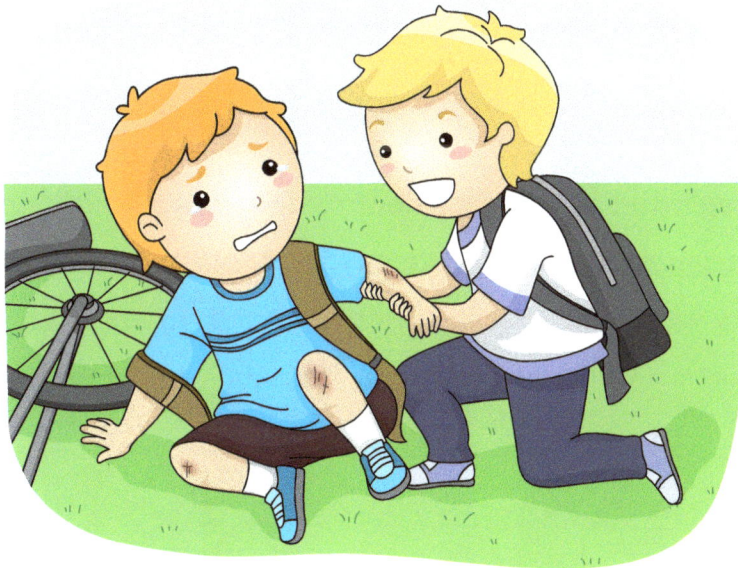

Children who are attempting to avoid vestibular stimuli will be afraid of movement activities. They will be fearful on playground equipment. They dislike being picked up and they appear to be clumsy or uncoordinated. You may notice they avoid the stairs or hold tightly to the rail, perhaps with both hands.

Those who are seeking vestibular stimulation are unable to sit still. They need to be in constant motion. They fidget, rock, and spin. You will notice them to be impulsive, and they crave movement. Every place they go they run instead of walk. They are risk takers both inside the building and out. They love to be upside down, and like to hang backward off a couch or chair.

Good strategies for children with vestibular issues are swinging, jumping on mini-trampolines, and riding trikes and rolling toys. They like spinning activities such as playing on a Sit-n-Spin.

KEY POINTS

- Some children are afraid of movement. They avoid playground equipment or stairs.
- They may not like to be picked up.
- Spinning activities, swinging, and jumping may be helpful.

Strategies to Teach Appropriate Response to Smells

The way a child responds to a sensory stimulus may sometimes need to be guided and taught. As his sensory perception begins to develop and become more mature, you can begin to teach him the proper response to a particular stimulus. A child who has never before realized that a flower actually smells good may now understand that the flower gives off a pleasant odor, but will not have the skill to communicate that thought. Model for him as you sniff the flower and smile then sniff it again. You might verbalize that the flower smells good, or indicate it by a simple manual sign. Gently teach him to respond to sensory stimuli the typical way or he runs the risk of fading into his own world more and more. In a kind way, offer him the replacement sensory activity when appropriate.

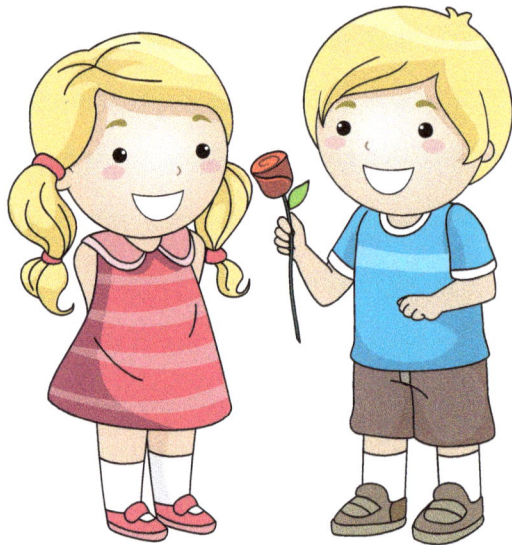

KEY POINTS

- Some children avoid aromas while others crave them.
- He will need to be taught about pleasant and offensive smells.

Strategies Concerning Self-stimulation

Self-stimulation is when a child feels the need to create stimuli or sensory input for himself. This often comes in the form of rocking, spinning, or hand flapping. The list of self-stimulating behaviors is endless and can involve any of the child's senses. He may engage in these behaviors to provide needed sensory input to himself, or as a calming mechanism. If you notice a child self-stimming, offer him a replacement behavior. Give him something else to do which meets that need for stimulation or calming. Self-stimulation is considered to be a negative way to cope. If a child is allowed to engage in self-stimulating activities endlessly he risks moving more toward isolating behaviors. When you notice self-stimulation activities, engage the child in sensory activities. Sensory input and stimulation will encourage proper behaviors and lessen the need for self-stimulation.

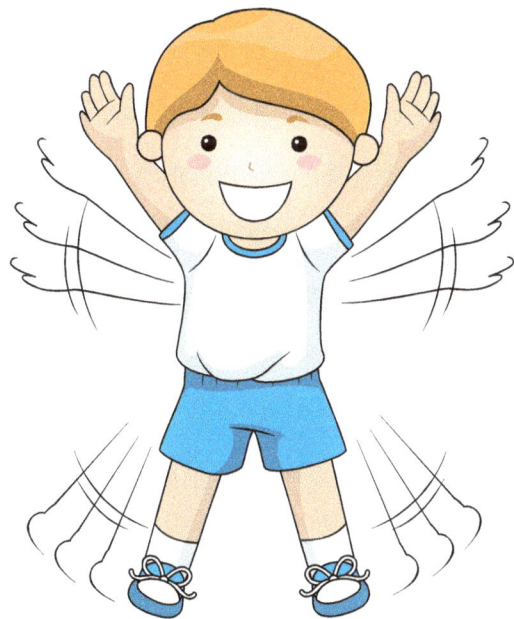

Observing your children will help you to notice any sensory needs they are displaying. Utilizing your ABC recording to observe and document behaviors more closely will enhance the classroom management. [6] A great teacher is one who recognizes the individual sensory needs of students and tries to accommodate those needs. Knowing that children with autism often have some sensory needs will help you plan for learning activities and anticipate potential difficulties.

⊶○ KEY POINTS

- Self stimulating activities such as rocking or hand flapping can be reduced by offering replacement activities.
- Self-stimulation activities are the result of the child seeking sensory input, or the child attempting to calm himself.

143

Strategies for Handling Anxiety

Children on the spectrum often display unusual anxieties or fears. Earlier we met Steven who was afraid of the erratic movement of butterflies. The idea of going outside when butterflies were present was very anxiety-producing for him. His teacher didn't share this same fear, but she understood that it was very real for him. Anxiety inducing situations may include such things as separation, vacuum cleaners, small dogs, eating in a restaurant or wearing a hat. Sometimes, we adults get frustrated when the anxiety triggers for children seem so silly and inconsequential to us, but we must remember how difficult it is for those children for whom the experience is really frightening. We need to take the fears seriously for the sake of the child and do what we can to lessen the anxiety.

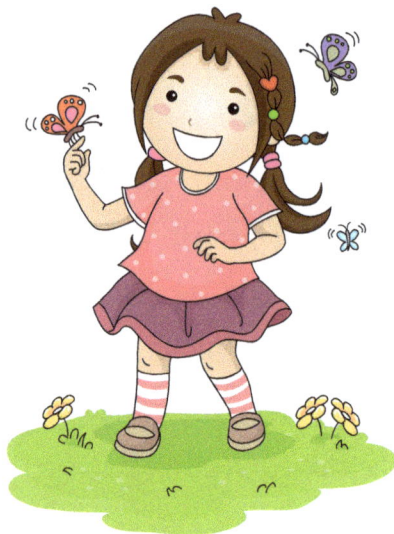

Some children may be able to build up a tolerance by being exposed to the stressor, such as a vacuum cleaner, in increasing increments of time or by starting at a far distance and coming closer in gradual increments. A visual timer may help a child see how long the stressor will be present, and knowing it will end may make it more tolerable. Three-year-old Jacob had major separation issues, and was helped by a picture of mom taped to the top of the timer during therapy sessions. He could see exactly how much "red" was left on the timer until he could see her again. Separation anxiety is sometimes helped by allowing the child to carry a photo puppet on a stick or a picture of the missed family member. Children benefit by cues to recognize when they are beginning to feel anxiety and to have a go-to plan of action to help control or reduce the anxiety. This might include use of a stimmy (something small to hold or rub), knowing how to take deep, calming breaths with eyes closed, or a calming statement that the child can repeat in times of stress.

Be sure to have a calm down place somewhere in your classroom-not a time out spot, but a location for a child to go when he senses he is about to become overwhelmed. Some teachers use aquariums in their classroom as a calming option, such as, "let's go watch the fish for a few minutes." The calming effect is exactly why some dentists have aquariums in their offices. Other teachers use a calm down bottle with a mixture of water, oil and glitter as a calming visual, stuffed animals to hug and hold, calming lotion that can be rubbed on arms or hands, a CD player with quiet music, or a small, soft blanket. Make sure the child understands he is not in trouble for using that spot, but is using that spot as a tool to help him cope.

Strategies for Managing Meltdowns

Despite a positive environment, great relationships, developmentally appropriate teaching and all the best planning in the world, meltdowns will still happen. That's a promise. Remember the difference between a tantrum and a meltdown. While the tantrum is over when the child gets his way and it requires an audience, a meltdown can go on and on. A child in the middle of a meltdown has no concern for his own safety, and may not even be aware of his environment, including your presence. By the time a child has reached this point he is no longer able to respond to his environment or to you. The child is completely out of control and is on sensory overload. You will feel the same way. The child needs you to recognize his loss of control, and needs your help to regain it, but most of the time won't be able to verbalize it. Once the child is in meltdown mode, your options are limited. Keep the child safe. Don't try to reason with the child because, at that point, he is beyond reason. Watch out for chairs that can be thrown, glass doors that can be kicked or other children who can be harmed. If a meltdown sometimes happens in your classroom, have a plan in which the other children can be calmly moved to another location for a few minutes, if need be. All they need to be told in a calm voice is "We are going to give Tyson a chance to calm himself down. Let's give him a little privacy." An adult will need to just remain with the child who is having the meltdown until it runs its course.

With a young child, if you see the meltdown is imminent (and as a good observer, you will get to recognize the signs and triggers for that particular child) distraction with a preferred toy or other item or activity may work, and help the child regain control before it's too late. Some children can actually recognize the feeling and alert you when a meltdown is coming. As a nonverbal preschooler, Nicole would look at adults with panic in her eyes and sign, "Help me! Help me!" as she began to feel the meltdown approaching. However, most little ones cannot identify the feelings of growing sensory overload. With an older child, you may be able to quietly remind him to calm himself, whether with a particular phrase, deep breaths, or a firm touch. The child does not enjoy the meltdown any more than you do. When the meltdown is over, you will probably both be exhausted, and that may not be the best time to try to converse. A very young child most likely is not developmentally able to recall and talk about more positive options for behavior next time––an older child might. If you do have a conversation about the meltdown, talk about other options for handling sensory overload or stress. Visuals may help to demonstrate other options.

🔑 KEY POINTS

- Meltdowns will happen, caused by sensory overload.
- Safety of all the children is your primary goal as the meltdown runs its course.
- You cannot reason with a child having a meltdown.
- A meltdown differs from a temper tantrum.

Those Terrible Tantrums

Tantrums are triggered by a child either wanting something or wanting to avoid something. The preschooler may want a specific toy, specific person, or time with a certain preferred activity. He may be trying to avoid a task, person or situation. A child having a tantrum typically has a goal in mind and if that goal is reached, the tantrum stops. The child may first try other means to get his needs met, and when that doesn't work, the tantrum is the next step as a play for power. In trying to avoid a tantrum, do acknowledge that you know what the child wants without giving in, and then move on. "I know you want more cookies, but you had two and snack time is over. Now, would you like Play Doh or cars?" A child having a tantrum wants an audience because he is hoping that someone in the audience will eventually meet his demand, so if he loses the audience, the tantrum usually ends.

Tantrums don't usually last long and are very situation specific, as opposed to meltdowns which can go on for a hour or more. The tantrum may involve crying, screaming, stomping and jumping, and lying on the floor and kicking. It's not pretty. Often you can see a tantrum coming as the child escalates. Sometimes you can find a way to distract a very young child and sometimes with an older child a little humor can actually stop the escalation enough that the child is able to find a more appropriate way to ask for what he wants. If a child does escalate into a full blown tantrum, calmly hold your ground. As long as safety is not a concern, simply ignore the behavior. Withdraw all attention, and remember negative attention is still attention. That means no talking, no looking at the child, no acknowledging what is happening. Don't fall into the trap of feeling you must keep talking, because the child isn't listening anyway. The worst thing to do is give in and give the child what he is asking for.

Behavioral experts will tell you that intermittent reinforcement is the most powerful kind. In other words, if a child has a tantrum and succeeds in getting what he wants even once in awhile, a tantrum is still a successful strategy for him. If, on the other hand, a child never gets what he wants by having a tantrum, that strategy is no longer a successful one, and will probably be discarded after several tries. The tantrum will end quickly if the child gets what he wants (which is why tired people give in) or finally just wears himself out. At that point, the natural inclination is to want to rehash everything that just happened. That

147

may not be productive when you are both tired and stressed. It's more productive to practice negotiation skills and problem solving as situations arise on a daily basis. The child needs to learn more successful strategies to get what he wants. Help him understand he will not get what he wants every single time he asks. Start early and start young to teach the child that he may hear "not today, that's okay" or something similar. State your position and then move on quickly to something else. Tantrums are one way a young child learns about the rules of the world and finds out the limits of his power. A tantrum is actually a step on the road to learning successful social skills.

Self-Regulation is the ability to understand and manage our own behavior when presented with various stimuli. This skill begins to develop rapidly in the toddler and preschool years. Self-regulation allows kids to manage their emotions when faced with stressful situations. Teaching strategies such as breath control and self-talk in advance of a meltdown will give the child a resource to call upon when faced with a stressful situation likely to trigger and unwanted behavior. After the child has learned calming techniques, the teacher may talk the child through the meltdown with verbal cuing. A teacher will want to model the act of self-regulating as a teaching technique by remaining warm and supportive in a challenging situation.

🔑 KEY POINTS

- Tantrums are goal driven.
- Tantrums require an audience to continue, so withdraw attention.
- Acknowledge the child's desire, then move on.
- Hold your ground as long as safety is not an issue.
- Help the child understand that he will not get what he wants every time.
- Help the child find more appropriate ways to work toward his goals.

It's
No
Biggie!

PART FOUR
RESOURCES

Chapter 9
Collaborate with Your Team

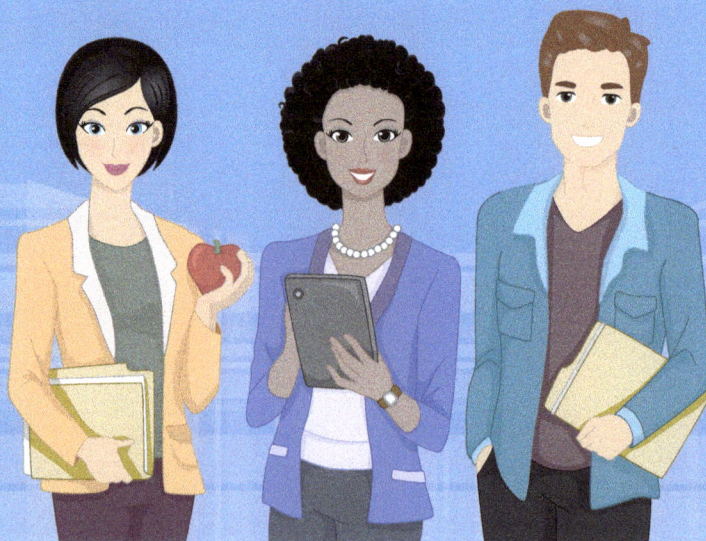

If you are working with a child within the public schools,
including children with special needs, you will have access to a team of providers. Working with a child with autism can be complicated and you need to work together with the service team to provide the most comprehensive and effective treatment plan. The makeup of the team will vary according to the individual child's needs. Work together with the parent to assemble a good team of skilled providers.

The most important relationship is that between the parent and the teacher. Both will have a profound effect on the life of this child. Work to form a strong bond with the parent from the first day. That bond is based on mutual respect and communication. Some parent-teacher pairs prefer to send daily communication books back and forth, or simply send notes each day informing the other of the child's successes and challenges for the day. Others prefer a quick email as time permits to compare notes. Even Facebook private messages have become an accepted tool. There are apps and programs such as Learning Genie that allow you to communicate electronic information to parents throughout the day. It is important to have some form of daily communication. Be sure to note good things that the child has done as well and problems that cropped up during the day. Whatever communication system you use with the parent, let that system work for you.

The special education teacher is responsible for coordinating with other professionals in the child's life. Although the makeup of each child's team will differ, there will be some common members. You will work closely with professionals in the medical and the educational fields.

One of the most important people on the team is the diagnostician. Even though the actual duties and even the title may vary state to state, the main responsibility is the educational testing and interpreting those tests. If needed, they are people who can provide behavior management suggestions and further resources.

Many school districts or states provide a BCBA (Board Certified Behavior Analyst) or an ABA consultant (Applied Behavior Analysis). You may work with a BCaBA, which stands for Board Certified Assistant Behavior Analyst. These professionals conduct behavioral assessments for children on the autism spectrum and help plan the educational program.

The SLP, or speech-language pathologist, is a crucial member of your team. This professional can assess deficits in various area of speech and language. The SLP will be a valued resource for you.

Occupational therapists (OT) can help you with sensory integration, fine motor skills and self-help skills, such as feeding and dressing. If your child is overly sensitive or lacks a sensitivity in any of the senses, this can lead to a variety of issues. The OT can help you design a program to remediate the problem.

The physical therapist (PT) does not deal directly with the issue of autism, but many of these children have concomitant medical issues which can benefit from the help of a PT.

Don't forget the importance of seeing the parent as a team member. As a teacher, the first step in working with a child should always be to talk with the parents. They know their child better than anyone, and they know what has worked at home and in previous child care settings. Find out what is motivating, or *reinforcing*, to the child, and what the child's special interests are. Ask what the child's sensory needs are, any particular fears, and if there is any time of day that is harder than another (with most young children, late afternoon is not so good). Any parent is going to be thrilled that a teacher is taking the time to contact them and to get to know their child better. This helps to establish a positive working relationship with the family, and allows you to be more comfortable when you need to contact the family again at some point in the future.

If you are working with a child who you are concerned about, but is not yet (and may never be!) identified as having special needs, it gets a little trickier. You will not have access to the team of providers if the child is not receiving direct services. The parent, however, will be a great source of information about what tricks and strategies work at home to obtain compliance, any sensory issues you should be aware of, and what is reinforcing to the child. This information will make a huge difference to you in the classroom. If the child goes through the evaluation process at any point, ask the parents to keep you informed about the process, and be ready to help in any way needed by the diagnostic team. Local agencies that are involved with autism and inclusion may be able to give you general advice that would be helpful. Never hesitate to start making phone calls to ask people to point you in the right direction for more guidance and education in working with special needs students and students on the spectrum.

🔑 KEY POINTS

- Know the team members and work together.
- The parent is an important member of the team.
- Create a daily communication system between you and the parent/ guardian.

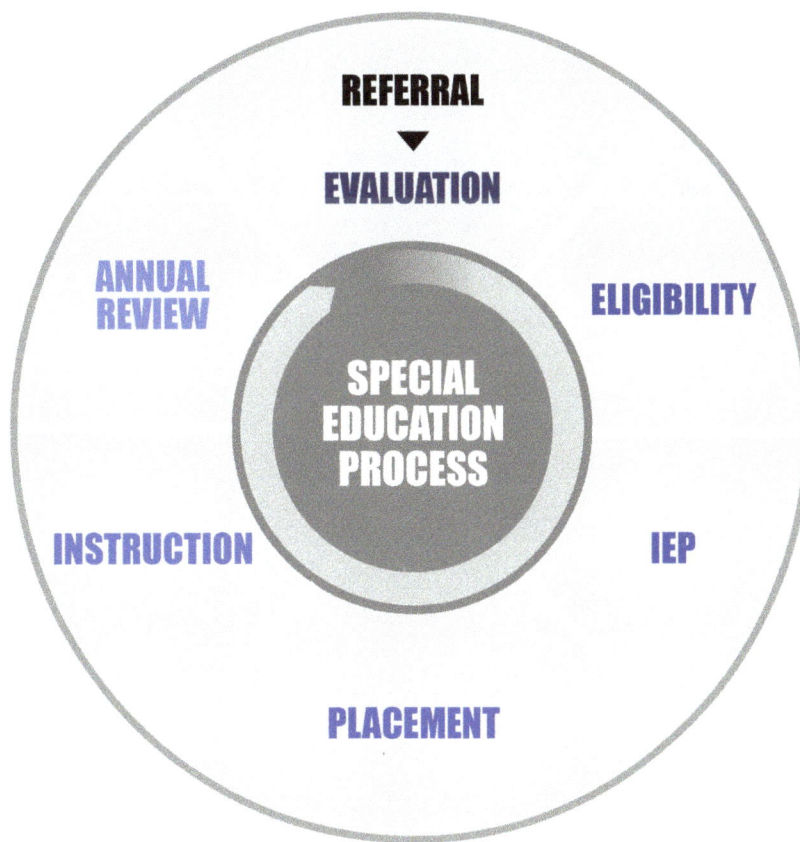

REFERRAL
▼
EVALUATION

ANNUAL REVIEW

ELIGIBILITY

SPECIAL EDUCATION PROCESS

INSTRUCTION

IEP

PLACEMENT

Chapter 10

Embrace the Process

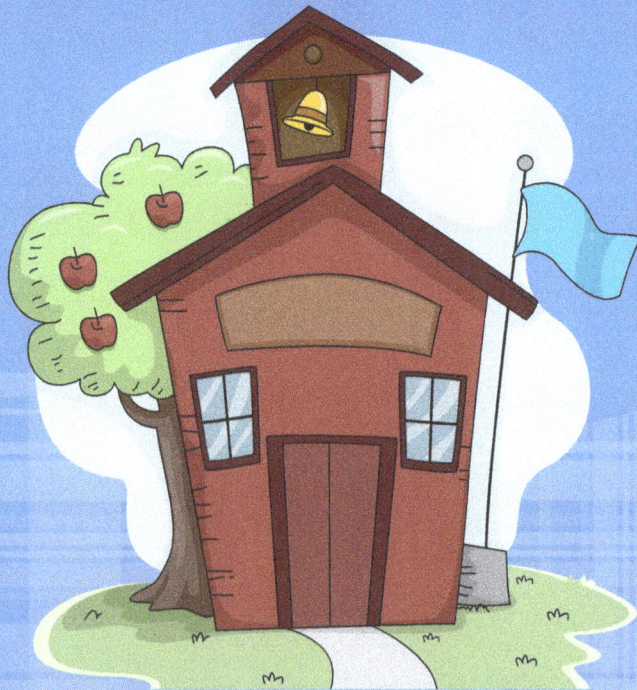

There was a time in the not too distant past when children with special needs were excluded from public school and from many child care centers. Now, all children with disabilities are guaranteed a free and appropriate public education in the least restrictive environment in the public school setting through IDEA- The Individuals with Disabilities in Education Act, passed in 1975. Children younger than three years old are provided special services through a state agency that is charged with finding and serving children who may qualify for those very early services. The names of these early child-find agencies may vary from state to state. These therapy services may begin shortly after birth for those students that qualify. Often if a baby is premature or is born with certain known medical or genetic conditions, the referral is automatically done by the pediatrician or hospital. Then, when the child turns three, he may begin to receive services through the public school system.

You will have children in your classroom who already have a diagnosis and a team of therapists and care providers in place. You might have children who you suspect may have a disability. You may have a child who is going through the diagnostic process while in your class. Regardless, it's important for you to have a working knowledge of the basics of the special education process. If you are teaching a child who is being served by an IEP, you are an important part of the team. If you are teaching a child who is going through the evaluation process, you may be asked to provide information on what you see in the classroom to help the IEP team make decisions about eligibility, goals and placement.

The basic steps are:

1. Referral: Parents and teachers are able to refer children for a special education evaluation based on their concerns, pediatrician concern, concerns from child care personnel, etc. Typically, the school district or child-find agency will determine any disability based on the parent report and determine whether an evaluation is necessary. Often the first step is to give parents and teachers what are called "alternative intervention strategies"- tips and tricks to try to determine if they might help a child achieve before looking further at special education services. In some cases, those alternative interventions may be waived if the concerns are significant enough. If a child is identified as possibly needing special education services, the student will be evaluated. The teacher's first step in the referral process is to discuss this with the parent. If the parent gives permission, the teacher can pursue the referral process.

2. Evaluation: Some parents may opt for private evaluation services that they pay for; the school district will also provide an evaluation for free. Only areas of concern will be evaluated. The evaluation results will be used to determined the child's eligibility for special services. Parent and teacher input is an important part of the evaluation process. Re-evaluation is conducted every three years to determine whether a child continues to qualify for services.

3. Eligibility Determination: The evaluation team determines, based on the results of the evaluation, whether or not the child meets eligibility criteria for special education services. The team will decide if this child qualifies as a "child with a disability" under the federal definition that is a part of the Individuals with Disabilities Education Act (IDEA) and these results may be shared with the parents.

4. IEP: If the child is found eligible for special education services, the team will then write the Individual Education Plan (IEP) that defines the types of services and amount provided. Special services fall on a continuum based on the needs of the child. Services may include physical therapy, occupational therapy, speech and/or language therapy and academic or pre-academic services provided by a special education teacher. An IEP is considered a legally binding document for the school district. An IEP can be modified or revised at any time by the team (for example, if goals or services need to be changed) and is written for a year at a time.

5. Placement: After looking at the goals for the child and the types of services needed, the most appropriate placement is determined. Does the child need to be served in a special education classroom for the majority of the day, or can the child attend regular classes with some pull out special services? Can a preschooler be successful in a typical preschool program or is an early childhood special education classroom more appropriate? How long should the school day be for this child? Is the child eligible for special services over the summer? Placement may be revised again at each subsequent IEP meeting, and if that initial placement doesn't seem to be working, it can always be changed at a specially scheduled IEP meeting.

The least restrictive environment clause (LRE) in special education means that a child will receive no more special education services than are actually needed. Special needs students are always encouraged to be a part of the regular education setting as much as is possible. Part of the special education process involves finding that right balance of services and regular education.

Instruction: The IEP goals are addressed by the designated providers with support from regular education teachers. Progress reports are provided to parents, just like a school report card.

Annual Review: The IEP is reviewed yearly. All members of the IEP team, including parents and regular education teachers (such as child care providers) have input as to the current functioning of the child, progress toward goals and what the next steps will be. New goals will be written based on the child's functioning and what members of the team observe.

While some students will receive services only through the public schools, others may receive services through a variety of public and private agencies or medical facilities. Some parents may opt only for the private and agency services. While the school system provides early services for qualifying students, parents are not required to access those services prior to mandatory school attendance age. It is a choice for each parent to make. Of course, we do know that early intervention is key!

⚿ KEY POINTS

- You may have children in your class who have special needs that have not yet been formally diagnosed.
- Never "diagnose" a child yourself.
- Parents may refer a child for evaluation if disabilities are suspected.
- An IEP is a legally binding document and must be followed in the public school setting. In private settings, following the IEP is considered best practice.

Chapter 11

Gather Your Resources

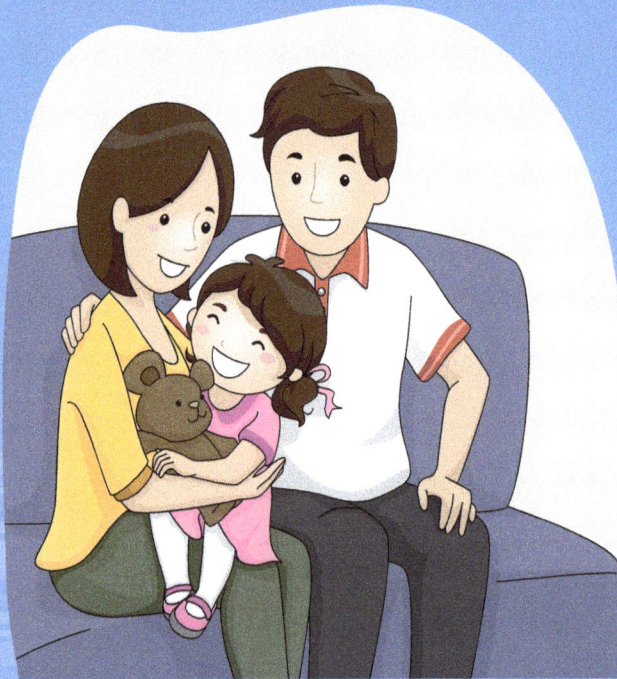

Resources are any opportunities that may be available

to you to better serve your students. Think about programs, therapies, materials, equipment or opportunities that you may be able to access. Networking with other teachers is a great way to learn what is available. Many resources look good but are beyond your limited budget. Ask other teachers about pooling resources, sharing resources, or making things that you see commercially available.

Check your school library for children's books such as *Albert is My Friend,* by Luck and Barboa. The Albert series is available in four languages. [11] Supplement this with the theme based unit guide available from TeachersPayTeachers.com at a minimal cost. *We Are all Stars* by Datema helps children learn to accept differences in others. [12] If you want to learn more about autism from a parent's point of view, or from the perspective of other teachers, read *Stars in Her Eyes: Navigating the Maze of Childhood Autism* by Barboa and Obrey.

If your program is operated by a public school system or is funded by the government you will have access to a support system. The most important resource you have available to you is the IEP. The Individual Educational Program is built just for that specific child based on formal and informal testing and observation of the child. This testing should define the child's strengths and challenges. Use that knowledge to teach the child in the way he learns best. The IEP is your roadmap guiding you to helping this child grow academically and socially.

Whether or not the child is in a public school or other government sponsored setting, you have resources you can tap. Each state has a Resource Center system. Although every state has this system, it may vary somewhat from state to state. Do a little research to see what your state offers. The National Educational Association (NEA), a teacher's organization, offers a variety of resources. You can access them online for a list of the methods and instructional materials they suggest. Even web resources such as Pinterest.com or TeachersPayTeachers.com have materials to meet your needs. Other formal autism associations have teaching resources available online.

One online resource that can be incredibly helpful to you is YappGuru.com. YappGuru.com provides you with reviews about educational apps that are commercially available on other sites. YappGuru.com is easy to use and allows you to investigate apps you may be interested in before you purchase them. This allows you to spend your money wisely. If there is an app that you are interested in purchasing, you can go to YappGuru.com and read reviews by experts and see what ratings other teachers have assigned to that app. The detailed reviews provide creative teaching ideas for educators using that app. Just enter keywords to find apps to meet your needs. You will need to register to access some of the features, but the registration is free.

KEY POINTS

- *Resources are any materials, therapies, programs or equipment that can assist you in teaching.*
- *Pool resources with other teachers to stretch your budget.*
- *Take advantage of books that contain helpful information to boost your teaching skills.*
- *Tap sources available through local agencies and governmental offices.*
- *YappGuru.com is a free resource to help you find appropriate apps to use in teaching.*

Glossary

Learn the Lingo

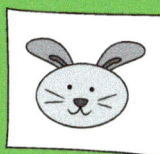

Rabbit

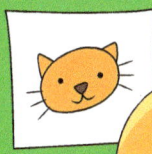

Cat

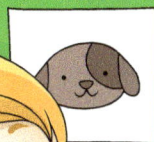

Dog

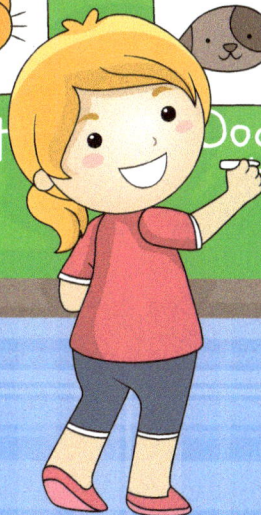

When working with children with special needs, you will encounter a whole new vocabulary. Acronyms are plentiful and confusing. Here are some common terms you may come across, along with their definitions:

AACs are augmentative and alternative communication devices for speech and language. This can refer to anything from a picture board to an advanced electronic device.

Abstract thinking may be difficult for people on the autism spectrum. While concrete thinking just deals with facts, abstract thinking requires a deeper level of thought or problem solving.

ABA is Applied Behavior Analysis, is a highly structured systematic program that has been proven to be an effective way to teach children with autism.

Action rhymes are a favorite teaching technique. Pairing actions with oral language helps develop language skills.

ADA is the Americans with Disabilities Act which assures civil rights protections to all persons with disabilities.

ADD stands for Attention Deficit Disorder. ADD may occur along with autism, or may stand alone.

ADHD is Attention Deficit Hyperactivity Disorder, which is basically ADD with hyperactivity added.

Alerting stimulants will encourage children to attend to a given activity. These stimulants are the opposite of the activities that calm a child.

Allergies and food sensitivities are common in children with autism. Certain foods or environmental elements can ramp up the activity level beyond control, or may make the child lethargic or even ill.

Apraxia is difficulty in completing motor movements. Oral apraxia results in severe difficulties with speech and should be treated by a licensed speech-language pathologist.

Aroma therapy may be beneficial as some smells may invigorate and others may calm a child. Smells have been shown to stimulate memory.

Articulation is the way a child pronounces his words.

Attachment to an object is common in autism. The child becomes overly- attached to a toy, a stuffed animal, or even a random object. He finds comfort in that object.

ASD is a shorter way of saying autism spectrum disorder.

ASL stands for American Sign Language. We normally don't teach true ASL to nonverbal children with autism, but rather more simplified signs which align better with our English system of grammar.

Asperger's Syndrome is recognized by the child's awkwardness in social situations but it does not impede his language skills, except social communication. The new physicians' medical terminology includes Asperger's in the classification of autism, but you will often hear the term used to delineate the difference between this and classic autism.

Aspie is an affectionate term for a person who displays Asperger's Syndrome.

Audiologist is a licensed professional who tests hearing.

Auditory is the sense of hearing.

Auditory processing is the way the brain interprets what the ears hear.

Auditory sensitivities are common in children with autism. A child may be too sensitive to sounds, or not sensitive enough to sounds.

Autism in its classic form is characterized by deficits in both social interactions and communication. It includes hypersensitivity and hyposensitivity to stimuli from the environment.

Avoidance behavior is a coping mechanism employed by many children with autism. Avoidance is characterized by the child tuning out, or even physically removing himself from a situation.

Babbling is the production of early speech sounds such as "bababa." It is a normal step in a child's development at about 6 months of age.

Biomedical treatments address the physical symptoms of children on the spectrum. The goal of biomedical treatments is usually to address the psychological symptoms of the disorder such as autism.

BIP, or Behavior Intervention Plan, is a plan created by the teacher and therapists to manage behavior. It becomes part of the IEP, and therefore is a legally binding document in the public school system.

Body language is a part of communication that does not come naturally for children with autism. You will need to teach what various facial movements indicate, as well as what body stances should indicate to him. Body language includes eye contact, facial expressions, postures, and other bodily factors that affect communication.

CDD is childhood disintegrative disease where a child develops normally until about age two, then regresses and shows characteristics of autism.

Choice board is one type of visual aid which you can make. Use pictures or small objects to present a visual array of objects from which your child may choose at a specific time.

ChoicesChats© are short simple talks you have with the child to discuss the choice he has just made and what alternate choices may have been more appropriate.

Cognitive impairment is difficulty remembering, learning new things, problem solving, concentrating, or making decisions in everyday life. Cognitive impairment ranges from mild to severe. This used to be referred to as mental retardation, a term which is no longer acceptable.

Co-morbidities are other diagnoses that may accompany a primary diagnosis.

Constructive play is happening when the child is making something with blocks or other materials.

Cue is a signal, either verbal or nonverbal that you give the child. You may cue him that it is turn to do something, or may cue him for an answer to a question. A cue may also be known as a prompt.

Cycling is common in the development of children with autism. They may learn a skill, regress, and re-learn it. If the child is cycling, don't give up. Teach and re-teach as needed. Each time a skill is re-learned it should take less training.

Deep pressure refers to the use of weighted blankets, vests, or firm massage. This is a useful therapy technique applied under the direction of the OT.

Descriptive praise is being specific when you praise the child. Tell him exactly what he did well as opposed to the vague words such as, "Good job!"

Desensitization is used to teach the nervous system to react less to a certain stimulus. The offending substance is presented in graduated amounts, slowly increasing as the child acclimates to it.

Discrete Trial Training is a formal, structured program of teaching which breaks skills down into small steps. Teachers who want to use this system must be trained in the technique to use it appropriately.

Dysgraphia is a learning disability that affects a person's ability to write.

Early Acceptance Education© is a term coined by Dr. Barboa and Jan Luck to denote teaching tolerance of diversity to young children. Early acceptance can reduce bullying in later years as the children become friends at a young age despite their physical or mental differences.

Echolalia is the repetition of a word, phrase, or sound that the child has heard from someone else. Echolalia may be immediately after he hears the stimulus or may occur much later, which is known as delayed echolalia.

Expansion is a language enhancing strategy wherein the teacher repeats a sentence or phrase uttered by the child and lengthens it. For example, if the child says, "Daddy go," the teacher can expand that to, "Daddy goes to work and you come to school."

Expressive language is the language a person produces.

Facilitated communication happens when a teacher assists the child to touch pictures to show his wants and needs.

FAPE stands for Free and Appropriate Public Education. Every child, regardless of disability, is entitled to a free and appropriate public education.

Flapping is a sensory stimulant characterized by the child flapping his arms. Your OT can help you replace this behavior with a more appropriate way to meet his sensory needs.

Functional play is when a child plays appropriately with a toy, as opposed to just staring at it or watching the parts move or spin.

Generalization is when a child learns something, then applies it to other situations. Sometimes children may generalize inappropriately, such as calling all men "Daddy," while other times generalization is a valuable skill allowing carry-over of learning.

Gesture is any bodily movement that helps the child understand what you are trying to communicate to him. Often a hand movement, it could be a facial gesture, head movement or other.

Gluten is a protein that is present in some grains. Some children with autism appear to benefit from a gluten free diet.

Guided access is a setting on the iPad which gives teachers and parents control over the child's use of the device. It will allow you to control the apps and programs that the child may access.

Gustatory refers to the sense of taste.

Hand leading is simply the child taking your hand to lead you to a desired object. You should strive to replace hand leading with a higher level of communication.

Hand-over-hand is a method of teaching a child by placing your hand over the child's hand to guide it while completing tasks.

Hyperacusis is an abnormally high sensitivity to sound.

Hyperlexia is a term to describe a skill wherein the child demonstrates a special ability to "call words" or to read words verbally at a higher level than he can understand.

Hypersensitive means overly sensitive in any of the senses.

Hyposensitive means that particular sense is deficient.

IEP stands for Individualized Education Plan (or sometimes Program). Having this document in place is what determines the difference between regular education and special education. After a child has been tested and is determined eligible for special education services, this is the document that spells out type and amount of services provided, placement and specific goals, among other items. The IEP is individualized, meaning that it is written specifically for a particular child. An IEP is considered a legal document; the terms of the IEP are mandatory. If you teach a child who has an IEP, you be able to get a copy of the IEP from the parent, or, with parental permission, from the school district itself. As someone who teaches the child, you are considered a part of the IEP team.

IDEA is the Individuals with Disabilities Education Act. This federal law assures a free and appropriate education for all children, including those with disabilities.

Inclusion is providing educational services within the regular education setting to a child who has special needs.

Indirect requests are statements given to a person in hopes that he will understand that you are actually asking him to perform an action. For example, if you say, "Your face is dirty," what you really mean is, "Wash your face."

Interoception is the process of understanding signals from the body like breathing, hunger, pain, or the need to go to the toilet or sleep.

Jargon is commonly known as baby talk. It is a normal stage in early speech development (about 6 months of age).

Joint attention is the communication between two people as they interact. Many children with autism do not display age appropriate joint interaction with another person.

Journaling is a helpful technique for teachers in early intervention classes. Journaling will help you track student progress and is helpful in communicating with the parent.

LEA refers to the local education agency, such as the local public school. He may attend a private school or child care center, but the LEA refers to the public school which is responsible to provide his services.

Learned helplessness is a phenomenon that happens when we help a child too much with his activities and he fails to learn to do things for himself at a normal level.

Learning style refers to the way that the child best processes information. Some people learn better through the visual sense and others learn better through the auditory. Most children learn optimally through touching and doing.

Light cozies are rectangular pieces of material with magnets along the edges which can be attached to fluorescent lights to soften the light in the room. Cozies are commercially available and should not be home made due to fire hazard.

Literal thinking describes the way many people with autism think. They take your words very literally.

LRE, or the least restrictive environment is the placement that best enables a child to meet his needs while giving him no more special education services that are necessary. The child should be served with typically developing peers as much as possible and should receive no more special education services than are needed for the child to meet his potential.

Mainstreaming is the process of integrating a child with special needs into a regular classroom for part or all of a school day.

Manding refers to the instruction giving to a child. Manding can take the form of pointing or asking.

Modeling is one of the strongest teaching techniques you possess. Show the child the behaviors you expect through your own actions.

Olfactory refers to the sense of smell.

Open ended questions are questions that require more than one word to answer.

OT is short for occupational therapy, which deals with fine motor control and functional use of the hands; an occupational therapist may be part of an IEP team. The ultimate goal of an OT is to help the person achieve independence in his life. Therapies are usually sensory based.

Overgeneralization is when a child "over-learns" a word or concept. A child who has just learned to say, "Dada" may use that term to refer to all men.

Parallel play is seen when the child plays alongside another child, each largely playing independently of the other. At times they may imitate each other or briefly interact, but that is limited.

PDD stands for pervasive developmental disorder. A child with PDD is considered to be on the higher end of the spectrum, and often goes undiagnosed.

PECS® stands for Picture Exchange Communication System©. This highly structured program requires special training and uses small pictures to facilitate communication.

Perseveration is repetition of a sound, word or activity.

Phonological processes is the term used when a child struggles with a certain class of speech sounds, as opposed to just one sound.

Pica is eating non-edible objects. This is fairly common in children with autism and it must be controlled.

Pragmatics is the social aspect of language. Children with Asperger's struggle with the pragmatics of language, but not with expressive or receptive skills. Examples of pragmatics include social greetings, idioms, and maintaining a conversation.

PrepChats© are a simple, short chat you have with your child to prepare him for a situation that is coming up. For certain events you will have the same chat repeatedly.

Pretend play is commonly called "make believe." This is known as symbolic play.

Prompt is a cue or a signal you give the child to help him know it is his turn or to help him know what to do or say next.

Proprioception refers to the sensory system that lets the child know where his body is in relation to the space around him.

PT is short for physical therapy, which deals with the large muscles of the body, balance, and navigating the environment. A physical therapist may be part of an IEP team.

QR Codes are patches or tags developed by an organization called "If I Need Help," which can be scanned to obtain important information in case a child is lost. The patches are registered online and can be scanned by smartphones.

Receptive language is the language that the child understands, as opposed to the language he can actually produce.

Reinforcers are rewards given to a child to modify behavior of any type.

Rephrasing is a technique for teaching language. When a child produces a sentence that contains language errors, simply rephrase the sentence using the correct grammar. For example, if he says, "Her wants candy," reply, "Yes, *she* wants candy."

Respite is care or funding provided to the family to provide care for the child in the absence of the parent.

Rett's Disorder is a rare genetic disorder that resembles the behaviors seen in autism.

Role playing is a simple technique to allow the child to rehearse the skills needed in a social situation.

Rote memory is pure memorization. A child may count by rote memory but not be able to count objects.

Scaffolding is a term used to describe assistance that you provide to a child to enable him to complete a task. You will find the child's strengths and build on those skills.

Scripting is memorization of something he has heard and can repeat back verbatim. This is often non-functional, and while it may seem cute it interferes with real communication.

Self-regulation is the ability to understand and manage your behavior and your reactions to things happening around you.

Self-stimulation is the phenomenon of a child creating stimuli for himself. Common types of self stimming behaviors are flapping, humming, spinning, or rocking.

Sensory integration is processing sensory information that your body receives.

Sensory processing is the neurological process that organizes sensation from one's own body and the environment, for effective functioning. Sensory processing includes what we feel, see, hear, touch and taste. Sensory processing disorder refers to significant concerns with the ability to process sensory information.

Sign is a hand movement that represents a word. The sign may be taken from a formal system such as American Sign Language, or may be modified for the child.

SLP stands for speech-language pathologist. The SLP deals with both the sounds that are produced to make words (speech) and putting the words together to communicate (language). A speech-language pathologist may be part of an IEP team.

Social referencing is when the child looks to others to acknowledge his accomplishments. A child with autism often lacks this desire.

Splinter skills are skills that a child has which are far above his other abilities.

Spontaneous speech is the speech that a child generates on his own.

Symbolic thought occurs when the child realizes that a picture or object actually represents a real object.

Tactile is the sense of touch.

Tactile Defensiveness is shown by behavioral and emotional responses, which are aversive, negative and out of proportion, to certain types of tactile or touch stimuli that most people would find to be non-painful, neutral or pleasurable. In young children, extreme tactile defensiveness may inhibit their ability to participate in daily activities or activities at school. Tactile defensiveness is the avoidance of touch.

Task analysis is breaking a task down into smaller steps.

Token system is a reward system where tokens are given as rewards for a task or behavior. Tokens may be exchanged for another greater reward.

Vestibular sense allows the child to understand where his body is in relation to the earth.

Visual refers to the sense of sight.

Visual cues remind a child of what he is to do. Visual cues may be pictures, printed words or objects.

Withdrawal is a coping strategy seen in children with autism. If we do not help the child with autism learn appropriate coping techniques, there is a very real danger that he will retreat further and further into his own world.

Footnotes

1. NAEYC. (2009). Early Childhood Inclusion. 2-3. http://www.naeyc.org/files/naeyc/file/positions/DEC_NAEYC_EC_updatedKS.pdf

2. http://www.cdc.gov/datastatistics/

3. (2016) "Identified Prevalence of Autism Spectrum Disorder," http://www.cdc.gov/ncbddd/autism/data.html

4. Webster, D. (2016) Goodreads. https://www.goodreads.com/quotes/66493-if-all-my-possessions-were-taken-from-me-with-one

5. Obrey, E. & Barboa, L. Tic Toc Autism Clock: A Guide to Your 24/7 Plan, Hendersonville, Tennessee: Goldminds Publishing, 2014

6. Bijou,S., PetersonR., & Ault, M. (1968). A method to integrate descriptive and experimental field studies at the level of data and empirical concepts. Journal of Applied Behavioral Analysis. Summer; 1(2): 175–191.

7. Vygotsky, L. S. (1978). Mind in society: The development of higher psychological processes. Cambridge, MA: Harvard University Press

8. NAEYC,(1998).Two-Way Communication hppt://www.naeyc.org/familyengagement/principles/2

9. , W. "Helping Parents Deal with the Fact That Their Child Has a Disability." CEC Today, Vol 3. No. 5. The Council for Exceptional Children.

10. Skinner, B. F. (1953). Science and Human Behavior. SimonandSchuster.com

11. Luck, J. & Barboa, L. (2015). Albert is my Friend: Helping Children Understand Autism. Hendersonville, Tennessee: Goldminds Publishing

12. Datema, M. (2016). We are all Stars. Hendersonville, Tennessee: Goldminds Publishing

13. "The Picture Exchange Communication System." http:www.autism-society.org/living-with-autism/treatment-options/pecs.

14. "The Note." Seinfeld. Fox. WNYW, New York City. 18 Set. 1991.Television.

15. Agassi, M. (2014). Hands Are Not for Hitting. Minneapolis, MN: Free Spirit Publishing.

16. Agassi, M. (2004). Words Are Not for Hurting. Minneapolis, MN: Free Spirit Publishing.

17. Havighurst, R. (1952). Human Development and Education, 3d ed. David McKay Company, Inc., a division of Random House, New York. N.Y.

18. Hannaford, C. (2013). Smart Moves, 2nd Ed. Salt Lake City, Utah: Great River Books.

19. Gilbreth, F.B. (1911) Motion Study. Van Nostrand: Princeton, NJ.

Parting Words

We hope you find the information in this book to be helpful. Our purpose in creating this book is to reach out to you, the teacher, who is trying hard to teach all children well and make a difference in their lives. Your job is so important and often thankless. It is demanding and difficult. Adding children with special needs into the equation magnifies the challenge. The surge in the incidence of children with autism has not been reflected in the training offered to most teachers of early childhood programs. Our intent is that by giving you some basic educational principles supplemented by the basics of autism, we can reduce the teaching burden. This knowledge should allow you to have fun every day and love your job as passionately as you thought you would when you signed your contract.

The key to bringing the successful teaching process into focus is to always remember that the most important person in the whole educational process is the child. That statement is no less true when regarding the child with special needs. Each child is a growing person deserving of respect and dignity. The child is the heart of the education process. As teachers, we advocate for all children. As you learn to observe the children carefully to determine possible causes of behavior, you will be taking the steps to guide them to more socially acceptable behaviors. Only when the academic behaviors are in place, is learning possible.

The real learning and enhanced child development come from the generous giving of time and engagement. With patience, open minds move mountains, and open hearts change lives. It's all about building relationships and trust. Think of the power inherent in that reality. The amazing effect that you have on so many young lives every day, every hour. Each word from your mouth, each glance that you give has more impact than you can even imagine.

The great writer Maya Angelou once said, "I've learned that people will forget what you said, people will forget what you did, but people will never forget how you made them feel." Our challenge to you today is to instill in each child a joyful heart that allows them to be lifelong learners. Teach with love and you will find yourself loving to teach. Take a deep breath, relax, and remember Dustin's mantra, "It's no biggie!"

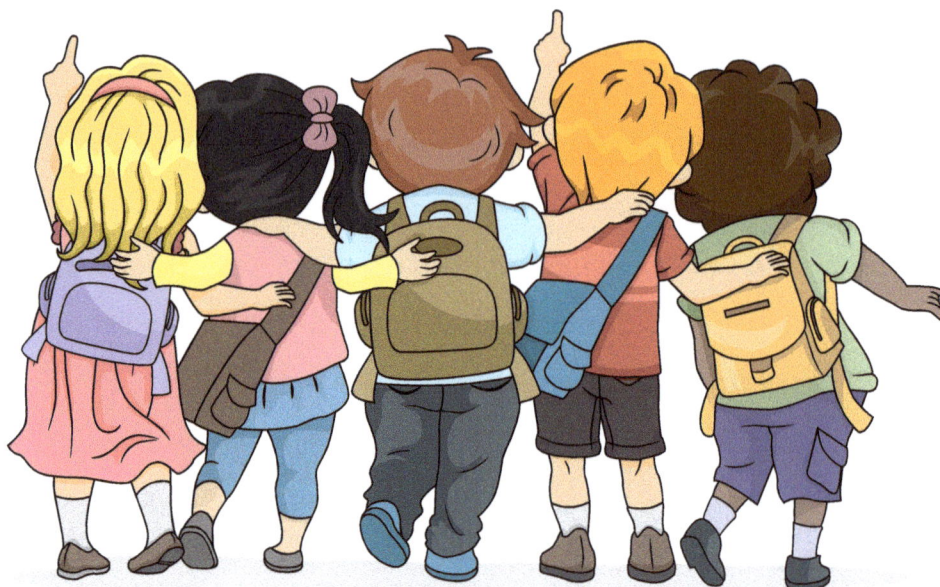